VITAMIN
E

VITAMIN E

Your Protection Against

Exercise Fatigue,

Weakened Immunity,

Heart Disease,

Cancer, Aging,

Diabetic Damage,

Environmental Toxins

RUTH WINTER, M. S.

THREE RIVERS PRESS • NEW YORK

Copyright © 1998 by Ruth Winter

Published by Three Rivers Press, a division of Crown Publishers, Inc., 201 East 50th Street, New York, New York 10022. Member of the Crown Publishing Group.

Random House, Inc. New York, Toronto, London, Sydney, Auckland
http://www.randomhouse.com/

THREE RIVERS PRESS and colophon are trademarks of Crown Publishers, Inc.

Printed in the United States of America

Library of Congress Cataloging-in-Publication Data
Winter, Ruth, 1930–
Vitamin E : your protection against exercise fatigue, weakened immunity, heart disease, cancer, aging, diabetic damage, environmental toxins / by Ruth Winter
p.   cm.
Includes bibliographical references (p.).
1. Vitamin E—Physiological effect.   2. Vitamin E—Therapeutic use.   I. Title.
QP772.T6W54   1998
612.3'99—dc21   97-15955
CIP

ISBN 0-609-80132-5

10 9 8 7 6 5 4 3 2 1

First Edition

CONTENTS

INTRODUCTION

VITAMIN E, YOUR GREAT PROTECTOR

Vitamin E's history has been fraught with promise and despair. It has never achieved the acceptance of its cousins A, B, C, and D. For more than half a century after its discovery, it remained an enigma—the center of an intriguing scientific controversy.

Naysayers claimed that a vitamin E deficiency disease had not been proven in humans, and treatment with vitamin E was worthless. They called it "the shady lady of nutrition" or "the vitamin in search of a disease."

The U.S. Food and Drug Administration for years officially denied vitamin E had any therapeutic value. Yet the FDA official who once read me a statement to that effect, when asked afterward, "What do you really think about it?" admitted to me that he took vitamin E each day before jogging.

The shady lady has at last become highly respectable. Scientific evidence concerning vitamin E's many benefits is rapidly developing.

The results of recent epidemiological studies have heralded the benefits of vitamin E and other antioxidant nutrients. For example:

- A U.S. study of women nurses found those with high intakes of vitamin E had a 34 percent lower risk of heart disease.[1]
- Nutrition intervention trials in Linxian County, China, associated a reduced risk of several types of cancer, especially stomach cancer, with dietary supplements of vitamin E, beta-carotene, and selenium.[2]
- Studies show that the risk of cataract may be reduced by 40 to 50 percent with dietary supplements of vitamin E and vitamin C.[3]

Vitamin E is, according to the latest scientific reports, one of the most effective preventative substances against heart disease, cancer, and some of the disabilities associated with aging. In fact, the president of the American Heart Association in 1996 declared vitamin E one of the biggest advances in cardiology. Cancer specialists and neurologists are issuing report after report that vitamin E is effective in warding off some malignancies and nerve damage.[4]

Why did it take so long for recognition of the value of this vitamin? Even before the positive results from recent major studies, physicians and other intelligent individuals began swallowing their doses of vitamin E. They began to believe that what the "food faddists" and "health nuts" have been saying all along may be absolutely true—vitamin E is of great benefit to the human body and, in medicinal doses, may help prevent and treat many of our major physical ailments.

Is vitamin E necessary to your health? This book is an attempt to inform you about the fascinating history and current scientific excitement about vitamin E, the inexpensive, formerly unappreciated, vital vitamin.

1

THE DISCOVERY

Why did female rats given a diet of rancid lard conceive young in a normal manner but fail to carry to term? What was it in lettuce that could correct the fertility problem? The year was 1922, and two young American scientists, Dr. Herbert M. Evans and Dr. Katherine S. Bishop, wanted to find out. Their aim was to determine whether reproduction was dependent on "some nutritive substance different from those which produced growth and adulthood."[1]

At first, Drs. Evans and Bishop thought that the vitamin C in lettuce cured the rat mothers' problem, but then they determined only the oil of the vegetable worked. To their amazement, they then discovered that wheat also cured the infertility.

Intrigued, Dr. Evans went to a nearby flour mill and saw "three great streams flowing from the milling of wheat berry; the first constituted the outer cover or chaff; the second, the endosperm—the white so-called flour; and the third, which came in flattened flakes, stuck into such units by its oil content—the germ."

Dr. Evans found that "single daily drops of the golden yellow wheat germ oil proved remedial."

The substance in the lettuce oil and the wheat germ was vitamin E.

To obtain a proper scientific name for their discovery, Dr. Evans consulted George Calhoun, a professor of Greek at the University of California at Berkeley.

"What does the substance do?" Calhoun asked.

"It permits animals to bear offspring," Evans replied.

So Calhoun took *tokos,* the Greek word for childbirth, and the Greek verb *pherein,* meaning to bring forth, and the suffix *ol* for alcohol; thus vitamin E was named tocopherol.

It is now accepted that there are four tocopherols and four closely related compounds, tocotrienols, in the E family. Tocopherols are widespread in nature. They are in almost all plants and animals so far examined. The most active of them found so far is alpha tocopherol. All the tocopherols have been synthesized and are readily available. The different forms of vitamin E have unique stability and biochemical activity. They may vary in their potency and their potential benefit.

Vitamin E is fat soluble—it dissolves in fat, but not in water. It is highly concentrated in the adrenal glands, found above the kidney. The adrenals regulate sodium and potassium in the blood, produce certain sex hormones, and help the body respond to stress.

The lack of sufficient vitamin E causes dramatic and sometimes peculiar ailments in animals. Reproductive failure and muscular dystrophy are seen in many species. The first detectable sign of tocopherol deficiency in the rat and in the monkey is the fragility of red blood cells. In the chick, it is encephalomalacia, a degenerative brain disease. The first organ affected in the turkey is the gizzard. In the calf, the first sign of vitamin E deficiency may be sudden death from heart failure.

As startling as the vitamin E deficiency symptoms are in animals, for more than thirty years a physical effect could not be proved in humans. There were many claims for almost every tissue of the body, but no disease was definitely associated with vitamin E, such as the beriberi of vitamin B, the scurvy of vitamin C, or the night blindness of vitamin A.

Then, in 1952, using a newly developed laboratory test, Dr. Paul Gyorgy and his associates at the University of Pennsylvania, showed that the blood of vitamin E deficient babies was particularly prone to hemolysis, a weakness of the red blood cells that causes them to rupture easily.[2]

In 1966, researchers at St. Luke's Hospital in New York City reported in the *American Journal of Clinical Nutrition* that premature infants fed a formula containing polyunsaturated cottonseed oil as the source of fat showed irritability, edema (water retention), skin lesions, and changes in the red blood cells. When vitamin E was administered, the symptoms cleared.[3]

In 1968, two more cases of hemolytic anemia in newborn infants fed commercial formulas were reported. Dr. Max Horwitt of the University of Illinois cited a fourteen-month-old baby fed cottonseed oil intravenously for nineteen days before death. The baby had cerebellitis, a brain condition almost identical to the encephalomalacia of vitamin E deficient chicks.

Such findings led the American Academy of Pediatrics to recommend for the first time, in 1967, a minimum level of 0.3 IU (international units) of vitamin E per 100 kilocalories in infant formulas.

The study that set the first adult vitamin E standards was conducted by the University of Illinois's Dr. Horwitt under the auspices of the National Research Council's Food and Nutrition Board, the branch of the National Academy of Sciences that sets official recommended daily requirements. Dr. Horwitt put adult men at Elgin State Hospital, Elgin, Illinois, on a diet low in vitamin E and with varying amounts of polyunsaturated fats (PUFA). After a year or so, the vitamin E levels in their blood fell slowly, and the first physical sign of deficiency began to appear: an increased fragility of red blood cells. The more PUFA the men ate, the greater their symptoms.[4]

Dr. Horwitt also noticed that a large percentage of the men developed peptic ulcers. He attributed this to the irritating effect of oxidized fat and pointed out that many people are adversely affected by fat-fried foods.

Fearful of producing irreversible damage, Dr. Horwitt induced only mild vitamin E deficiency in his subjects. Yet his results were dramatic enough to make the Food and Nutrition Board of the National Academy of Sciences set, in 1968, a minimum daily requirement for vitamin E at 30 IU. The board recommends the government standards for the recommended daily intakes (RDIs) of nutrients. This amount was intended to allow for a moderately increased consumption of polyunsaturated fatty acids, which deplete vitamin E.

Dr. Denham Harman, Professor of Biochemistry at the University of Nebraska, pointed out that experimental evidence showed the incidence of breast cancer in female mice increased with both the amount and degree of unsaturation in their diet of fat. This finding, he said, agrees with the observation that free radicals caused by such things as ionizing radiation may contribute to tumor development. He said other experiments have shown the incidence of mammary cancer induced in female white rats by cancer-causing agents was higher when the rats' diet contained 20 percent (by weight) corn oil, an unsaturated fat, in comparison to those fed the same amount of coconut oil, a saturated fat.

"This may explain why," he continued, "the high incidence of gastric carcinoma in Iceland and Japan may be related to the relatively large amounts of highly unsaturated fats consumed by this population. Similarly, in Sweden and other countries with a high consumption of fish, the death rate from stomach cancer in white males in the 55-to-64-year age group is two to three times as high as that of the comparable population in the United States."

The increase of polyunsaturates has taken place with the emphasis on lowering cholesterol. Polyunsaturates are from vegetable sources and are liquid at room temperature. Saturated fats, which are from animals and contain cholesterol, are usually solid at room temperature.

In 1989, the Food and Nutrition Board nevertheless decided to reset the recommendation for vitamin E at 15 IU for adult males and 12 IU for adult females. The theory was that 30 IU was much more than could be ingested in the daily diet and that 15 IU was sufficient to prevent vitamin E deficiency.

The RDA for vitamin E is an object of controversy among nutritional scientists. Some point out that until 1968 there were no daily requirements set for vitamin E. Does that mean that before 1968 we had no need of vitamin E? Or is it that scientists just learned that we do indeed need it?

Many nutritional experts now recognize marginal or subclinical vitamin deficiencies may exist. In this condition, vitamin status is poor (depleted reserves or localized deficiencies) but with no overt symptoms of a deficiency.[5] In a U.S. study, for example, subclinical vitamin deficiencies were reported in groups of schoolchildren, elderly people, neonates, and mothers at the time of delivery. It is now believed by many scientists that chronic marginal vitamin deficiencies may reduce resistance to environmental toxins and carcinogens. They also suggest that chronic marginal micronutrient status harms physical performance,[6] immune function, and mental behavior.[7]

We were told for years that vitamin E is so abundant in our food supply that it is virtually impossible for a deficiency to be present. We now have to ask, is vitamin E degraded in products we get from the market? Does processing, freezing, or cooking destroy it? Is there such a thing as a vitamin E deficiency?

In actuality, there are more questions than answers about the shady lady of nutrition. Do we know enough about vitamin E requirements to detect the symptoms of vitamin E deficiency? Is vitamin E being measured accurately in the human body and in human food? Is vitamin E being given therapeutically in its most potent form? Is vitamin E really needed to maintain health?

Dr. Horwitt, at eighty-five years old, confessed to the *Wall Street Journal* in 1993 that he was taking vitamin E. For decades, he had railed against what he called "the overfeeding of vitamins" to credulous, pill-happy Americans.[8]

"I'm ashamed to do it," he told the *Wall Street Journal*'s David Stipp, "because of my attitude toward taking vitamins. But an explosion of studies show that vitamin E is a possible preventative for heart disease, cancer, and dozens of other disorders."

This book attempts to inform you about research concerning vitamin E and comments on such work by experts. You will then have to make a decision, preferably with professional advice, whether you should increase your intake of vitamin E.

2

THE SHADY LADY FIGHTS YOUR

FREE RADICALS

One of the biggest benefits of vitamin E, as you will read throughout this book, is its ability to fight free radicals.

What are free radicals? They are not former Communists, although they are kind of immoral. They are molecules that are "single" and looking for partners and are not unlike a dangerous person who may answer an ad in a singles publication. They look for a mate by stealing someone else's partner or by attaching themselves to a couple. Just like the "other" woman or man, they cause a lot of disturbances and destroy relationships.

The most common and potentially hazardous free radicals are the oxygen "singles." We are oxygen-breathing animals and we cannot live without it, yet our cells are constantly traumatized by oxygen free radicals. They may deform and corrode any partner they touch.

Free radicals, like most antiheroes, do have their good side. They play a big part in our ability to kill microbes, and without them we would be helpless to break down food, twitch a muscle, think a thought, or reach for a vitamin pill. Free radicals are controlled with extraordinary precision by our bodies, and usually they are kept in line. It is only when we age or are under abnormal stress that free radicals escape their assigned duties and begin doing their dirty work on our cells. Environmental factors such as cigarette smoke and pollution seem to increase production of free radicals.

There is a large body of evidence—a great deal of which is described in this book—that free radicals can directly and indirectly

- damage fats within the cells
- fragment DNA strands, producing genetic mutations
- damage proteins, resulting in the loss of biological activity
- produce inflammation
- cause severe injury or cell death in the lungs
- damage blood vessels
- decrease the activity and availability of neurotransmitters (brain chemicals that carry messages from one nerve cell to another)
- change LDL (bad) cholesterol into artery-clogging substances
- promote cancer
- produce signs of aging such as wrinkles and deterioration of other organs
- contribute to the development of a number of conditions such as cataracts, arthritis, Parkinson's disease, and stroke[1]

Our defenses against out-of-control free radicals are the antioxidants manufactured in our bodies and the antioxidant vitamins taken in the diet and in supplements. Their job is to break down free radicals into water and oxygen (nonradical) through the action of various defensive enzymes and to reduce the concentration of radicals in the body with the help of free radical scavengers. For more than thirty years, scientists have known that vitamin E—a fat-soluble vitamin—can penetrate the fatty membrane of cells and remove dangerous oxygen "singles." With the aid of its partner, vitamin C—a water-soluble antioxidant that gets into the fluid compartments of cells—vitamin E helps reduce your body's burden of harmful free radicals.

As you will read in this book, vitamin E's ability as an antioxidant can do much to protect you against common ills such as heart disease, cancer, and other body and brain disrupters.

3

VITAMIN E AND YOUR BLOOD

Primitive humans knew that if blood was drained from the body, the body died. Yet only in the past generation has blood really begun to be understood by scientists, and only recently have they realized that vitamin E is essential to the health of red blood cells.

An adult has about ten to eleven pints of blood and some sixty thousand miles of vessels to contain it. Through these vessels, the blood carries oxygen from the lungs and nutrients from the intestinal tract to all body tissues. It also distributes heat produced by working muscles and, because of its water content and mobility, acts as a body-temperature regulator. It also guards against disease.

The normal amount of red blood cells that transport the oxygen for the body's tissues is 5–7 million per cubic milliliter for males and 4.5–5 million for females. At birth, the normal red cell count is slightly higher. By the second month, it falls to about 4 million and remains at that level for several months. It then rises to 4.5 million until puberty.

The average hematocrit (amount of red cells per total blood volume) is 47 percent in men and 42 percent in women. For the red blood cells to remain at the normal, healthy level, the cells that die off each day must be replaced by reticulocytes (new cells) released from the bone marrow. Since the normal life span of a red blood cell is approximately 120 days, $1/120$ of the total red cell mass, forty thousand to fifty thousand per cubic milliliter, must be replaced daily.

When there are not enough healthy red blood cells, the condition is called *anemia*. Symptoms of anemia may be irregular or absent menstruation, loss of libido, low-grade fever, heart failure, intestinal complaints, and jaundice. Many symptoms of severe anemia resemble those of acute blood loss. These encompass weakness, dizziness, headache, roaring or humming in the ears, spots before the eyes, fatigue, drowsiness, irritability, a false sense of euphoria, and psychosis.

Vitamin E deficiency causes anemia in many species and in different ways. In poultry, for example, vitamin E deficiency anemia causes the leaking of blood into tissues. In rodents, severe destruction of the red cells occurs only when vitamin E deficient animals are exposed to oxygen stress. In swine, the anemia is primarily the result of defective formation of red blood cells.

What about vitamin E anemia in humans?

It is difficult to experiment with vitamin E deficiency in people because of the possible adverse effects, but in another primate, the rhesus monkey, the results are dramatic.

Dr. Coy D. Fitch, professor of biochemistry, at the Department of Internal Medicine, St. Louis University School of Medicine reported at the International Symposium on Vitamin-Related Anemias in 1968 that simple vitamin E deficiency in young rhesus monkeys always ends with the animal's death from anemia. He described how he fed thirty-two young rhesus monkeys vitamin E deficient diets and thirty control monkeys the same diet with vitamin E supplementation.

"On routine examination, the vitamin E deficient monkeys appeared normal for five to thirty months and seemed to match the growth of their vitamin E supplemented counterparts," Dr. Fitch said. "Then, abruptly, there was rapidly progressive weight loss, excessive excretion of creatine necessary for muscle contractions, and anemia." The same devastating disease occurred in all the vitamin E deficient animals.

Dr. Fitch said he could not explain the variation in time of onset of the disease, but he found that it was unrelated to the level of vitamin E in the blood. He noted that vitamin E may be practically undetectable in the blood for two years before the onset of the disease.

In addition to the anemia and weight loss, Dr. Fitch found muscle weakness and wasting. But despite the rapid progression of the wasting, there was no evidence of muscle pain or tenderness, nor of coexisting neurological disease. Yet the monkeys became so weak they had to prop themselves up against their cage to stand. When they fell, they were unable to get up. Their skin tightened, and the contraction of the muscles surrounding their knees, hips, and elbows impeded their movement and hastened death.

Before death, there was a nearly complete wasting of the membrane enclosing the bowel, breathing became difficult, the heart rate slowed, and the mucous membranes turned white. There was swelling around the eyes, and sometimes jaundice. Even terminally, there was no diarrhea or evidence of heart failure, lung infection, or kidney disease. Just before death, the monkeys became cold and flaccid. Even if vitamin E was given, the disease was no longer reversible.

"The cause of the devastating symptoms in the monkeys," Dr. Fitch said, "was severe anemia."

Vitamin E deficiency anemia has been found in premature infants. Dr. Samuel Gross, Dr. David K. Melhorn, and Geraldine Childers, all of Case Western Reserve University in Cleveland, found that of 234 premature infants studied between 1968 and 1971, 80 percent had easily damaged red blood cells—and subnormal levels of vitamin E.

At birth, premature infants have iron stores approximating those of full-term infants; yet, because of their rapid growth in the first year of life, premature infants require more iron. To prevent iron-deficiency anemia, approximately three milligrams of elemental iron per kilogram of body weight per day is needed. However, achieving this level is often not feasible after they leave the hospital. Consequently, many hospital doctors give premature infants as much as twenty-five milligrams of iron during hospitalization (seven to ten days) in an attempt to anticipate need.

Dr. Gross and his colleagues found that giving big doses of iron to vitamin E deficient infants increased the damage to red blood cells. Furthermore, when iron and vitamin E were administered together, the absorption of both substances was impaired.

Red blood cells are responsible for carrying oxygen to various parts of the body. Both vitamin E and iron are necessary for the oxygen-carrying function of the blood. However, too much oxygen can damage the blood and other tissues, as pointed out earlier in this book. Premature infants put in 100 percent oxygen-filled incubators become blind.

Astronauts in the early space flights showed some blood changes after being in the high-oxygen atmosphere of the space capsule. They were given prophylactic vitamin E before ensuing flights. Patients who receive treatment in high-pressure oxygen chambers are also given vitamin E to ward off red cell oxygen damage.

Vitamin E deficiency evidently makes red blood cells more susceptible to damage from medications, such as iron, and from environmental stresses, such as too much oxygen. One theory is that oxygen free radicals make fat in the human body rancid. Once rancid fat deposits (lipid peroxides) are formed in the cell, there appears to be progressive damage to red blood cells, which swell and ultimately rupture. Increasing evidence suggests that the vitamin E levels in humans and animals affect the development of these rancid-fat deposits in the cell.

Can supplemental vitamin E, a natural antioxidant, protect our blood cells from damage by oxygen free radicals?

The answer may lie with the people who inherited *glucose phosphate dehydrogenase deficiency (G6PD)*. This genetic disorder causes red blood cells to be easily damaged by oxygen and the cells die off faster than normal. Significantly low levels of vitamin E have been found in these individuals. Administration of 800 IU per day of the nutrient over one year to patients with G6PD significantly improves their red blood cell life span and blood oxygen concentration.[1]

Another genetic disorder leading to fragile red blood cells is *sickle-cell anemia*. Most red blood cells are restored to their normal shape when exposed to oxygen, but in this inherited condition some remain irreversibly sickled. The more irreversibly sickled cells, the more severe the anemia. Sickle-cell patients have been found to have low levels of vitamin E, and their blood forms more oxygen free radicals.[2]

In a study in which sickle-cell patients were given 450 IU a day of vitamin E, there was a significant decrease in the percentage of their irreversibly sickled cells—from 25 percent pretreatment to 11 percent posttreatment.[3]

PREVENTING CLOTS

Platelets are small, colorless disks circulating in blood that play a part in clotting. They tend to gather at the site of injury. This leads to deposits of fibrin, a protein in the blood that entraps blood cells to form clots. Cholesterol also get halted at the site—all of which contributes to the plugging of blood vessels.[4] Platelet stickiness is a significant factor in the development of atherosclerosis and other vascular diseases. Vitamin E inhibits platelet aggregation and the production of hormonelike substances, *prostaglandins,* which further stimulate platelet pileup.

Evidence for vitamin E as a clot fighter has been shown in the laboratory.

Rats fed palm oil, which contains vitamin E, have a decreased tendency to develop platelet pileups.[5]

When rabbits were fed an artery-clogging fatty diet, their output of a natural substance that greatly inhibits platelet pileup, *prostacyclin,* was almost completely suppressed. When the bunnies were given vitamin E supplements, lo and behold, their anti-platelet-pileup prostacyclin-generating system in their arteries returned to normal.

What about humans eating fatty hamburgers and greasy snacks, which are said to clog our arteries? When adults were given a supplement of 400 IU vitamin E a day for four weeks, they had significant reduction in platelet pileup.[6]

Maury Breecher, MPH, Ph.D., a well-known science writer and coauthor with James Anderson, M.D., professor at the University of Kentucky, of *Dr. Anderson's Antioxidant Anti-Aging Health Program* (Carroll and Graf, 1996), said he saw this firsthand on his own body: "I take four hundred units of vitamin E in the morning and four hundred vitamin

E in late P.M. for its anti-platelet-clogging properties. I think it is better than the aspirin a day that many medical docs take. Since I am diabetic, I prick my fingers to test my blood-sugar levels two to four times a day. When *not* taking vitamin E, it is hard to get a good hanging drop of blood because my serum moves like sludge. Since taking vitamin E, self-testing for sugar levels is easier because my blood flows cleanly."

Dr. Breecher says he began taking vitamin E years ago to prevent heart disease and stroke after doing stories about early studies that indicated vitamin E offered those protections.[7]

Scientists have shown in the laboratory what Dr. Breecher observed personally.

Dr. Paul Dowd, a professor at the University of Pittsburgh, is a pioneer in the study of vitamin K, a nutrient routinely used as a clotting agent in surgical procedures and many other conditions. After deciphering how vitamin K starts the process, Dr. Dowd became curious about how vitamin E might interfere with it. In laboratory experiments using enzymes extracted from rat livers, Dr. Dowd and Barbara Zheng, a graduate student, showed that a by-product of vitamin E metabolism, *vitamin E quinone,* competes with vitamin K by effectively blocking the enzyme's ability to initiate clotting.[8]

"This understanding also reinforces the idea that people have to be careful about how much vitamin E they take," Dr. Dowd cautions. "Each person's metabolism is different, and some people may form more vitamin E quinone than others." An overload of vitamin E quinone could result in excessive bleeding or even trigger a hemorrhagic stroke.

Dr. Dowd was then more interested in exploring vitamin

E quinone's clot-inhibiting property. He explained that the anticoagulants now widely used act indirectly and slowly to inhibit clotting, while vitamin E quinone acts directly and possibly faster, which could save lives, time, and money when someone is in danger of forming life-threatening clots. For example, anticoagulants are used to prevent blood clots triggered by accidents or surgery, especially operations to repair a broken hip, replace a heart valve, or bypass a clogged coronary artery.

Vitamin E supplementation may also be important to women on birth control pills, who may have a risk of blood clots. Women on oral contraceptives who were found to have reduced vitamin E levels and increased platelet clotting were given 200 mg/day for two months. Following supplementation, blood samples from the women showed markedly reduced platelet activity (sticking together).[9]

WHEN BLOOD IS SHUT OFF

Free radicals also cause their mischief when blood flow is shut down either by an event such as a stroke or during heart surgery. Restoration of blood flow to previously blood-starved (ischemic) organs results in a rapid increase in oxygen free radical damage to cells. Animal studies have indicated that vitamin E is depleted when the blood flow is stopped and that supplemental vitamin E helps prevent free radical damage associated with blood cutoff and restoration. In patients with coronary artery disease undergoing heart-lung bypass, oxygen free radical damage has been noted. In such patients pretreated with vitamin E twelve hours before surgery, the number of their oxygen-damaged cells did not increase significantly during or after bypass surgery. In patients not pretreated with vitamin E twelve hours before surgery, there was a progressive increase in cell damage.[10]

Though there are many controversies about the effect of vitamin E on the human body, few could argue about its necessity for healthy blood.

4

VITAMIN E AND YOUR HEART

In the early 1970s when I was writing an article about vitamin E, I came across the work of two Canadian physician brothers who were reporting the good results they were obtaining giving vitamin E to heart patients.

The Shutes were maintaining that "vitamin E improves the ability of the body to utilize oxygen as no other physiological substance can" and that "it is relative insurance against blood clots, whether in the coronary artery or the brain or the leg. The use of vitamin E is simple, cheap, and safe. It never causes hemorrhage. It opens up unused blood vessels to give you detours around blocks you have in your circulation."

Being a trained newspaper reporter, I then went to the medical director of the American Heart Association, who, at that time, was Dr. Campbell Moses. He told me, "There is no proof that vitamin E has any effect on heart disease. Patients with heart disease who are on a downhill course will reach for straws. The Shute brothers are good doctors and give good, conventional treatment to their heart patients, in addition to vitamin E."

I then contacted Dr. Shute about Dr. Moses's observation, and in a letter he answered, "I was very interested in your quotation from the American Heart Association that the Shute brothers give 'good care,' although I don't know how they know. They have never seen us in action, and they have refused to send a committee up to look at our work. I wonder how they know what results we get, since they never look at them. And how do they know that people get results in our hands that can't be obtained in any other way? This is most amusing and silly. If we give good medical care and get corresponding results, is there no chance whatever that vitamin E plays any role in these results?

"Of course people shouldn't treat themselves," Dr. Shute continued in his letter. "There is real danger in this. Fortunately, the average patient has more to gain by treating himself than he has to lose by poor selection of a doctor. This is one reason why we have always been anxious to get this into medical hands. But, if medical hands continue to reject this, what alternative is there left but for patients to treat themselves, as they are doing by the hundreds of thousands?"

Twenty-four years after I received that letter from Dr. Shute and dutifully noted the opinion of the medical director of the American Heart Association, I was interested to read a news report: "The president of the American Heart Association stated vitamin E in either supplements or in food may help prevent heart disease and considered it one of the top ten research advances."

Jan Breslow, M.D., the American Heart Association president, had said in a year-end review of developments in the field, "Vitamin E appears to prevent coronary heart disease, a disease caused by fatty plaque clogging the arteries that feed the heart. Several studies in 1996 lend credence to this antioxidant vitamin's possible role in preventing heart disease.[1]

Ironically, the vitamin E study that stirred the most attention was called CHAOS—the Cambridge Heart Antioxidant Study.[2] It was designed to test the hypothesis that treatment with high doses of vitamin E would reduce the risk of myocardial infarction (MI), a heart attack caused by artery blockage. The British investigators selected 2,002 patients with confirmed coronary artery disease for a prospective, double-blind trial comparing vitamin E with a placebo. Half of the 2,002 men and women received the placebo. The other half was divided into two groups, one of which took 800 IU of vitamin E for two years, and the other, 400 IU for one year.

Vitamin E significantly reduced the risk of cardiovascular death and nonfatal heart attacks. Treatment did not affect serum cholesterol levels. Only eleven patients discontinued therapy because of diarrhea, heartburn, or rash, and risk of these side effects did not differ among the groups studied.

In just six months, the risk of nonfatal heart attack dropped 77 percent in both supplement groups. After a year and a half, all those who received vitamin E supplements had a quarter of the number of heart attacks as the control group, although there was an "insignificant slight excess of deaths from all causes in the vitamin E group (twenty-seven vs. twenty-three)."[3] Surprisingly, the 400 IU group did better than the 800 IU group.

The research concerning the connection between levels of vitamin E and heart disease is burgeoning. For example:

- Cross-cultural studies of sixteen European populations found a geographical correlation between low blood levels of vitamin E, and to a lesser extent vitamin C and carotenoids, and high rates of cardiovascular disease.[4]
- University of Minnesota School of Public Health's Dr. L. H. Kushi and his colleagues studied a group of more

than 34,000 postmenopausal women with no cardiovascular disease who in early 1986 completed a questionnaire that assessed, among other factors, their intake of vitamins A, E, and C from food sources and supplements. During the approximately seven years of follow-up (ending December 31, 1992), 242 of the women died of coronary heart disease. In analyses adjusted to age and dietary calories, vitamin E consumption appeared to be inversely associated with the risk of death from coronary heart disease.[5]

- The Health Professionals Follow-up Study tracked vitamin E use in 39,910 male health professionals, forty to seventy-five years old, for up to four years. The results were similar to the women's study. The men taking at least 100 IU of vitamin E had roughly 40 percent less risk of developing heart disease than those who took no vitamin E.[6]

Not all vitamin E heart studies have been so encouraging. Finnish researchers found no benefit, and some other researchers have had negative reports about the benefits of vitamin E as a preventative. Most recent reports, however, have been very positive.[7]

In a study of nineteen Western European and five non-European countries, researchers reporting in the *European Journal of Clinical Nutrition* did find positive results. They tracked premature mortality from coronary heart disease in men under sixty-five and related it to diet. The so-called French paradox concerns a diet high in fatty, rich food and a lower rate of heart disease than in the United States. These researchers concluded that "dietary alpha-tocopherol may provide at least as good an explanation as does wine for the paradoxically low rates of coronary heart disease in several European countries which have a relatively high saturated fatty acid intake."[8]

While there may still be controversy about the benefits of vitamin E in preventing heart disease, there is little disagreement about the state that most often leads to heart attacks and strokes—atherosclerosis. Atherosclerosis is a thickening and hardening of the walls of the arteries. The process usually begins with the deposit of fatty material such as cholesterol on the inner lining of the arterial wall. As more of these deposits form and increase in size, they gradually narrow the channel through which the blood flows.

Dr. Paul Dudley White, the father of modern cardiology, proclaimed in the early 1970s that atherosclerosis is "the great twentieth-century epidemic.[9]

"Arterial atherosclerosis involves the aorta, coronary circulation, cerebral circulation, and the circulation in the legs and kidneys," Dr. White said. "This disease—endemic throughout recorded history among the small percentage of the world's population rich enough to afford it—has in the past fifty years grown to gigantic proportions in the United States! Even worse, it is afflicting younger and younger men. In my practice in the past two months, I have seen five men under the age of forty so affected. The youngest was twenty-eight."

Most doctors now agree that all of us have some degree of atherosclerosis. How can vitamin E protect us from dangerously clogged arteries and blood vessels?

Cholesterol, despite its bad publicity, is necessary for our bodies. It is essential for producing new cells and manufacturing certain hormones. It is delivered throughout our systems by tiny packages made of fat and protein called *lipoproteins.* Lipoproteins are flat, disklike particles produced in the liver and intestines and released into the bloodstream. There are basically two major types, *high-density lipoproteins (HDLs)* and *low-density lipoproteins (LDLs)*. It is believed HDLs pick up cholesterol and bring it back to the liver for reprocessing. Some researchers believe HDLs may also remove excess cholesterol from fat-engorged cells, possibly even those in artery walls. Because HDLs clear cholesterol out of the system and high levels of it are associated with decreased risk of heart disease, HDL is often called good cholesterol. An LDL package, on the other hand, is considered bad because it drops its contents along artery walls as it travels from the liver to body cells.

The National Institutes of Health's National Cholesterol Education Program Guidelines say our total cholesterol should be below 200 mg/dl, LDL below 100 mg/dl, and HDL above 35 mg/dl. So it is not only the total amount of cholesterol in our blood that is important, but which lipoprotein package is carting it around.

One of the newer theories is that it is *not* high cholesterol or fatty substances in the blood alone that cause clogged arteries, heart attacks, and strokes—it is the oxidation—the rancidity—of that fat and LDL cholesterol. These substances are "bad" only when they become affected by oxygen.[10] Indeed, oxidized sites have been found in diseased arteries but not in normal arteries by researchers at the University of Washington, Seattle.[11]

Vitamin E deters LDL oxidation!

Dr. Ishwarlal Jialal, an associate professor of pathology and internal medicine at the University of Texas Southwestern Medical Center at Dallas, believes vitamin E packs a one-two punch in fighting heart disease. Not only does it inhibit the oxidation of bad cholesterol, the first step in atherosclero-

sis, it also impairs a second step—plaque produced by monocytes within the arteries.[12] The earliest sign of atherosclerosis
is the accumulation of *monocytes,* foamy white blood cells
filled with oxidized LDL cholesterol. These monocytes bind
to the lining of the arteries and secrete free radicals, which do
the oxygen damage and contribute to the development of the
blockage.

Dr. Jialal and his colleagues at Southwestern Medical Center reported in 1996 that they had done the first study that
shows that vitamin E helps to counteract monocyte formation
of plaque.[13]

The Texas researchers studied twenty-one healthy individuals before and after they took supplemental vitamin E
for eight weeks and again six weeks after they stopped taking
it. The last phase was included to compensate for the absence
of a placebo group.

The researchers found a decrease in free radicals by nearly
a half, a decrease of 20 to 35 percent in the binding of the
troublesome monocyte cells to the artery wall, and a 40 percent decrease in fat oxidation. Thus, this study provides novel
evidence of the effect of vitamin E within the cell to discour-
age monocytes from building blockages.[14]

Dr. Jialal believes this is a tremendous advance in the prevention of heart disease.

He says he does not recommend vitamin E for people at
large, but he does prescribe 400 IU of vitamin E for his heart
patients. He said when asked if he takes vitamin E, "I won't
answer that question."[15]

WHAT ELSE CAN VITAMIN E DO TO PROTECT OUR BLOOD VESSELS?

Atherosclerosis and spasms can obstruct the blood supply to the heart and blood vessels. The condition is called *ischemia*. Some epidemiologic studies have already shown an association between high dietary intake or high concentrations of vitamin E in blood and lower rates of ischemic heart disease, although others have not.

In chapter 3, it was pointed out that when ischemia—the loss of blood flow to a tissue—is followed by resupply of oxygenated blood (reperfusion), damage may occur to the tissues. During the final phase of bypass surgery, an operation to improve the blood flow to the heart, those devils, free radicals, form as surgeons briefly reflood the heart with richly oxygenated blood.

Dr. Terrence Yau of the University of Toronto has reported that vitamin E given before surgery improves the heart's ability to pump during the especially risky five-hour postoperative period. He and his colleagues base their conclusion on a study of fourteen people who took 300 mg of highly purified vitamin E every day for two weeks prior to their bypass operations and another fourteen bypass patients who received placebos.[16] Researchers at other institutions have reported vitamin E can protect against reperfusion injury.[17]

THE CHEST PAIN CALLED ANGINA

It is not surprising that vitamin E is being prescribed today for the treatment of *angina pectoris,* chest pain due to an insufficient supply of oxygen to the heart.

Japanese researchers discovered in a study of 110 people with angina that blood levels of vitamin E were significantly lower than in heart patients without angina. The authors concluded that people at risk for developing this chest pain might benefit from vitamin E in their diet.[18] A number of other studies in the United States and Europe have reported that the higher the blood levels of vitamin E, the lower the risk of angina.[19, 20]

LEG CRAMPS

Intermittent claudication also involves an inadequate blood supply, usually in the calf muscles of the leg while walking. It can also affect the buttocks, thighs, or hands. It is characterized by pain or tightening that occurs only after muscular exertion.

Dr. Knut Haeger of Sweden reported in the December 1968 issue of *Vascular Diseases,* an American medical journal, that he had been successful in treating cases of intermittent claudication with vitamin E.

"Some twenty years ago," he wrote, "encouraging reports on the use of vitamin E in the treatment of peripheral occlusive arterial disease were published simultaneously in several countries.…In 1953, the enthusiasm received a blow when a blind trial on forty-one intermittent claudication patients was assessed by exercise tests, clinical examination, and the patients' own opinions. The researchers were unable to demonstrate any difference between the patients treated with tocopherol and the untreated control patients."

He said that these tests were later criticized because the tocopherol preparation used was said to be inadequate.

He said he had seen results in his patients after only three months of medication and that it had later been observed it takes three or four months for the benefits of vitamin E to be manifested.

In Dr. Haeger's study, done in Malmö, Sweden, over seven years, 227 men were divided into four main therapeutic groups. They all had either peripheral occlusive arterial disease of the legs or intermittent claudication. One group was given vasodilator agents to dilate the blood vessels and increase the blood supply to the legs; another group was given anticoagulation treatment to keep the blood thin and clot-free; another group was given plain multivitamin therapy; and the fourth group was given alpha tocopherol.

The results were assessed on the basis of survival rate, amputation rate, subjective opinion of the patient, exercise tolerance test (walking distance to onset of pain), rate of healing of skin lesions, premature sick-pension rate, and in a limited number of cases, tests of vein function.

Dr. Haeger reported no significant difference between any of the therapeutic groups on survival rate, sick-pension rate, effect on skin lesions, and arterial flow measurements. However, significant differences were obtained in favor of vitamin E treatment regarding the patients' own opinion of the result, the walking distance, and the amputation rate. In those taking vitamin E, the average increase in walking distance was 150 percent as compared with 30 percent in those taking placebos.

The Swedish physician said, "The mode of action of tocopherol in arterial disease is still obscure. It is probable that the substance is active in the tissue metabolism and possibly acts as an adjunct in the better utilization of oxygen in the muscles....In animals we know two facts about tocopherol: it is, in some unknown way, involved in the oxidation systems of striated muscle; and deficiency of tocopherol leads to muscular degeneration. In patients with peripheral arterial disease, we have every reason to believe that, at least temporarily, the leg muscles work with an inadequate supply of oxygen, the normal metabolic system is damaged, and the normal enzymatic interplay is injured. It is conceivable that the addition of tocopherol may work towards a normalization of these processes."

A similar finding was discovered accidentally by Drs. Samuel Ayres and Richard Mihan of the University of California. They were experimenting with vitamin E in the treatment of rare skin diseases.

"One of the patients," the doctors wrote in *California Medicine* in 1969, "complained of severe night cramps until he began taking vitamin E. The doctors then gave vitamin E to twenty-four patients with leg cramps and to two with 'restless legs,' a condition where there is a sense of indescribable uneasiness, twitching, or restlessness that occurs in the legs after going to bed. In twenty-two of the twenty-six patients, the results were 90 to 100 percent effective. In the other four cases, the doctors reported moderately satisfactory results.

Dr. Haeger continued his studies with 300 mg/day vitamin E supplementation accompanied by a cessation of smoking and an increase in exercise. After two years the treated group had a 34 percent increase in arterial flow to the lower leg, with no change in controls receiving an anticoagulant or a blood-vessel-dilating medication. Patients' success in passing a distance walking test was 54 percent in vitamin E treated versus 23 percent in control subjects. In follow-up studies reported in 1982, similar results were obtained, according to Dr. Haeger.[21]

CAN VITAMIN E PROTECT AGAINST STROKES?

A stroke is a form of cardiovascular disease. So, just as it is important to keep blood vessels feeding the heart healthy, it is vital to keep blood vessels feeding and in the brain in good shape.

Stroke—the third-largest cause of death in the United States—occurs when part of the brain is damaged by not receiving a sufficient blood supply. There are several types of stroke:

- *Cerebral thrombosis,* the most common, occurs when a blood clot forms and blocks blood flow in an artery bringing blood to the brain. It usually develops in arteries damaged by atherosclerosis.
- *Cerebral embolus,* which also involves a block, but is usually caused by a wandering blood clot.
- *Subarachnoid hemorrhage* occurs when a blood vessel on the surface of the brain ruptures and bleeds into the space between the brain and the skull causing pressure on the brain.
- *Cerebral hemorrhage* is caused by a defective artery in the brain that bursts.

The many risk factors for stroke include:

- uncontrolled high blood pressure
- high cholesterol and high blood fat
- diabetes
- a strong family history of heart disease or stroke
- premature atherosclerosis from any cause

A common causes of stroke is a blockage in a carotid artery. One of these two major conveyors of blood to your brain lies on each side of your neck.

The National Institute of Neurological Disorders and Stroke (NINDS) of the National Institutes of Health is sponsoring the Asymptomatic Carotid Atherosclerosis Study (ACAS), a major multicenter prevention trial. One result reported thus far is that an operation to clean out the carotid artery in the neck is significantly better than any other medical treatment in preventing strokes.

Now the NINDS is sponsoring a major study of 3,600 patients at about thirty-six medical centers to determine if a healthy diet and common nutrients can prevent strokes from recurring. Dr. James F. Toole of Bowman Gray School of Medicine—the coordinating center—says that the trial is measuring whether the nutrients prevent second strokes or heart attacks in patients who have already had one mild, nondisabling stroke. The incidence of second stroke in patients who have had first strokes is between 7 and 10 percent per year. In addition, many first-stroke patients soon have a heart attack. Can both conditions be headed off by the nutrients? Dr. Toole says we will most likely know the answer in 1998 or 1999.[22]

Stephen Kritchevsky, Ph.D., of the division of Biostatistics and Epidemiology, Department of Preventive Medicine, University of Tennessee, and his colleagues have already studied the average carotid-artery wall thickness in 6,318 female and 4,989 male participants forty-five to sixty-four years old in the Atherosclerosis Risk Communities Study. They used a food-frequency questionnaire and correlated the answers with the thickness of the study participants' carotid arteries. They found, among men and women older than fifty-five, an inverse relationship between vitamin C intake and average artery wall thickness. An inverse relationship was also seen between wall thickness and vitamin E intake but was significant only in women. There was no such relationship between the antioxidant vitamins and wall thickness in persons less than fifty-five.[23]

The researchers concluded that there was limited support for the hypothesis that dietary vitamin C and vitamin E may protect against atherosclerotic disease, especially in persons older than fifty-five years.

DIABETES, TOO?

Diabetes mellitus is a common disorder. With insulin-dependent diabetes or Type I, which occurs mainly in young people, the pancreas produces little or no insulin. Type I accounts for 5–10 percent of diabetes. In non-insulin-dependent diabetes or Type II, people over forty are usually affected. Their insulin-producing cells in the pancreas function, but the output of insulin is inadequate for the body's needs. People who have this form are usually overweight. Type II accounts for 90–95 percent of diabetes and is nearing epidemic proportions due to an increased number of older Americans, and a greater prevalence of obesity and sedentary lifestyle.

Diabetics have a greater than average risk of developing atherosclerosis with its dangers of stroke, heart attack, and high blood pressure. People with diabetes are two to four times more likely to have heart disease, which is present in 75 percent of diabetes-related deaths (more than 77,000 annually). And they are two to four times more likely to suffer a stroke.[24] Therefore, if vitamin E can protect blood vessels, it may help diabetics avoid these potential consequences of their disease.

University of Texas Southwestern Medical Center at Dallas conducted a study of men and women with both Type I (insulin-dependent) and Type II (non-insulin-dependent) diabetes. Dr. Cindy Fuller and Dr. Ishwarlal Jialal and their colleagues chose to do the diabetes study, they said, because diabetics tend to have lower concentrations of antioxidants and to oxidize more bad cholesterol. Diabetics also experience greater protein glycation than nondiabetics. *Protein glycation* is the result of blood sugar binding to proteins. Diabetics typically have high blood sugar levels. If sugar binds to LDL, the bad cholesterol, it increases the buildup of blood-vessel-clogging plaque.[25]

The Southwesterners want to see if vitamin E could reduce LDL oxidation and decrease protein-sugar binding in diabetics.

Twenty-eight male and female insulin-dependent diabetics and non-insulin-dependent diabetics received either a placebo or 1,200 IU of vitamin E for eight weeks. Compared with the placebo group, the supplemented group had significant reductions in LDL oxidation. The benefit to LDL oxidation was seen in both types of diabetes, Dr. Jialal said.[26] However, there was no effect on the level of sugar-protein binding, they noted.

Dr. Jialal says that while he does not believe vitamin E has an effect on blood sugar, he believes there is a tremendous potential for it to prevent heart disease in diabetics.[27]

In another study, however, performed at the Universities of Liège in Belgium and Udine in Italy, vitamin E did reportedly reduce sugar-protein binding in diabetics. The diabetics in the study who did not receive the vitamin did not have the reduction.[28]

Vitamin E may also prevent damage to the retina, the light receptor cells in the back of the eye. Sven-Erik Bursell, Ph.D., of the Joslin Diabetes Center, Boston, found that diabetic patients have 16 percent less blood flow in the retina of the eye. In those receiving vitamin E supplementation, blood flow to their retinas became normal. This could conceivably slow or stop the development of retinopathy, he said.[29]

While the studies about vitamin E's influence on diabetes are still equivocal, in one study of elderly diabetics, patients given 900 mg/day of vitamin E supplementation showed mild improvement in blood sugar control.[30]

Can vitamin E help prevent diabetes?

Finnish researchers reported they took a random sample of 944 men aged forty-two to sixty who had no diabetes at the first examination. Four years later, forty-five of the men had developed diabetes.[31]

The Finns concluded that there was a "strong independent association between *low* vitamin E status before follow-up and an excess risk of diabetes at four years." They say this supports the theory that free radical stress has a role in the causation of non-insulin-dependent diabetes.

In addition to protecting against the damage caused by free radicals, the Finns believe that vitamin E may also help prevent diabetes by regulating *prostaglandins*—hormonelike substances—which play a part in opening and closing blood cells and by inhibiting potential blood clotting from platelet aggregation (see glossary).

HOW VITAMIN E MAY WORK

What if you are perfectly healthy and want to remain that way, but you can't pass up those burgers with fries and other fat-ladened treats? Can vitamin E come to your rescue? Maybe!

In a study, Gary Plotnick, M.D., and his colleagues at the University of Maryland Medical Center in Baltimore found that ingesting supplements of vitamin C and vitamin E can minimize the development of oxidative stress and its effects on blood vessels that occur after consuming a fatty meal.[32]

The Baltimore researchers measured the effects of vitamins C and E in twenty adults with desirable blood cholesterol levels (between 133 and 200 mg/dl). Each volunteer ate a nine-hundred-calorie meal that was 50 percent saturated fat. The scientists then measured blood flow in the people's forearm arteries within fifteen minutes of dining, and then every hour for six hours. They used an inflatable cuff to temporarily halt blood flow. Upon removing the cuff, they determined the degree to which the artery relaxed and widened to allow blood through.

Four hours after the fatty meals, the arteries had widened by only 8 percent, about half as much as they should have, Plotnick said. However, when the volunteers consumed 800 IU of vitamin E and one gram of vitamin C with the meal, the blood vessels widened and relaxed about 18 percent, which is about normal.

Though preliminary, these findings suggest that antioxidants might have a role in treating the effects of a high-fat diet, says Dr. Plotnick.

So, many exciting studies are being reported about vitamin E's beneficial effects on arteries, but is there a downside? Is there too much hype?

The CHAOS study, which attracted so much attention, had, among its results, "an insignificant excess" of deaths from all causes among its participants in the vitamin E group (twenty-seven versus twenty-three deaths).

Immediately, some researchers jumped on this, writing letters to the editor of *Lancet,* the British medical journal in which the study appeared.

One letter, from Farzin Fath-Ordoubadi, MRC, Clinical Sciences Centre, Royal Postgraduate Medical School, presented a theory about why heart attacks decreased in the CHAOS study but deaths increased. He speculated that the increased risk was seen early at the start of therapy and perhaps the vitamin E loosened some of the plaque and this caused the fatalities. He theorized that it might also be due to the combination of vitamin E and some medication being taken, including aspirin or another anticoagulant.[33]

Dr. Stephens, the lead author on the CHAOS study, said, concerning vitamin E contributing to the plaques breaking loose, that his group is awaiting data about chemical composition of the fatty plaques obtained at autopsies of those who died during the trials.

"Our instinct would be, however, that any excess early hazard is not due to excess plaque vulnerability to rupture. There were no differences in drug therapy between the patients who died early and the rest of the population," Dr. Stephens wrote.[34]

In another letter to the editor of *Lancet* concerning the CHAOS study, Dr. Kofo Ogunyankin of the University of California at Los Angeles School of Medicine considered the methodology of the study flawed. He wrote that systematic follow-up of patients was not maintained and that the authors relied on regional databases to determine heart attacks in patients.

"Since silent myocardial infarction [heart attack without noticed symptoms] could occur in up to 35 percent of these patients, and hence be unreported by patients, how reliable are the data on nonfatal myocardial infarction?" Dr. Ogunyankin asked.[35]

Dr. Stephens answered that there was no reason to believe that the outcome would be affected in a different way than in symptomatic myocardial infarction, and that his group did obtain 98 percent follow-up of patients at trial termination.

While the final chapter on the CHAOS and other studies showing vitamin E protects the heart and blood vessels is still to be written, many doctors are not waiting for those results.

Dr. Morris Brown, professor of medicine at Cambridge University and one of the researchers on the CHAOS study, said upon its publication, "Now we can confidently say that vitamin E protects against heart attacks. I will be recommending that patients with angina and those who are at risk of heart disease should be given supplementary vitamin E at a high dose."

Dr. Lester Packer, an expert in antioxidants at the University of California at Berkeley, emphasized that "the evidence on vitamin E is becoming more and more compelling with each well-done study, and the case for supplements is particularly strong. The evidence from studies using vitamin E supplements is stronger than that from studies based on dietary habits alone."[36]

Drs. Eric Rimm and M. J. Stampfer of the Harvard School of Public Health and researchers on the large Nurses Health Study and the Health Professionals Follow-up Study wrote in a review article in the *American Journal of Clinical Nutrition* about epidemiologic evidence for vitamin E in prevention of cardiovascular disease:

"Ecological studies of vitamin E have shown that regions

with relatively low dietary vitamin E tend to have higher rates of coronary heart disease, but it is difficult to adjust for other risk factors. Two large prospective studies found that persons who had used vitamin E supplements for more than two years had approximately 40 percent lower rates of CHD [coronary heart disease]. Short durations and doses less than 100 IU per day had no significant effect. The effect of dietary vitamin E was modest and nonsignificant. Adjustment for a wide array of other coronary risk factors had little effect on the findings, which were specific for vitamin E and not other supplements. The epidemiological evidence suggests that high doses of vitamin E may reduce the risk of CHD."[37]

WHAT ABOUT VITAMIN E IN YOUR DIET?

The American Heart Association's rationale, in addition to reducing the risk factor of obesity, was to reduce the amount of fat clogging the arteries. Cholesterol is the principal component of the atherosclerotic artery plugs. The AHA reasoned that by reducing the intake of cholesterol and other saturated fats in the diet, the amount of cholesterol in the blood would be reduced. When a fat is "saturated," it is usually an animal fat and is solid at room temperature. An unsaturated fat is usually a vegetable fat and is liquid at room temperature.

This diet theory is far from established fact, although many people are eating diets of polyunsaturated fats and skipping the cholesterol. Some studies performed by scientists have shown that men who have had heart attacks and then follow a low-cholesterol diet have fewer recurrent heart attacks. Other studies have shown that some populations that eat diets high in cholesterol rarely have heart attacks.

The Framingham, Massachusetts, heart disease study begun in 1950 initially included 5,209 residents of that town between the ages of thirty and sixty-two. Researchers have followed the participants for decades with support mainly from the National Institutes of Health. The pioneering study established that high blood pressure, high levels of blood cholesterol, cigarette smoking, high blood sugar, obesity, lack of exercise, and high levels of stress are more common among heart disease victims than among healthy people.

Many clinicians believe—and the Framingham study seems to bear it out—that people so inclined physiologically will manufacture cholesterol in their blood no matter what they eat.

Dr. White, the father of modern cardiology and a Massachusetts resident, attributed the increase in atherosclerosis to changes in lifestyles: "more calories, richer food, and more tobacco being consumed. With the disease already established, physical, emotional, dietary, or infectious stress can lead to complications such as coronary or cerebral thrombosis, or worse, sudden death."

The Shute brothers had an additional cause of the nation's high rate of heart disease. Dr. Wilfred Shute pointed out that prior to 1911, heart attacks were almost unknown. People had congestive heart failure (the heart is damaged by rheumatic fever, birth defects, or some other cause and cannot work properly) and strokes, but no fat-clogged coronary arteries. He maintains that in 1911 a new milling process was discovered and put into practice. The husk or hull on the wheat was removed and "white bread" came into being. The husk or hull is an excellent source of vitamin E for man.

If vitamin E does, indeed, protect the heart, then perhaps the diet of unsaturated fats recommended by the American

Heart Association could be harmful to the heart instead of helpful if it depletes the nutrient. Vitamin E is nature's own antioxidant. It keeps the fat from turning rancid. *Unsaturated* fats are more easily oxidized than *saturated* fats. Therefore, vitamin E is called into action more often when unsaturated fats are ingested than when saturated fats are ingested.

Dr. Max Horwitt, whose work at Elgin State Hospital set the standard for vitamin E daily requirements, reported this fact in 1961, and it has since been confirmed by many researchers. Virtually all vegetable oils contain tocopherols, but some, according to Dr. Horwitt and other researchers, contain insufficient quantities of the most active, alpha tocopherol, to counterbalance the effect of the polyunsaturated fats. The consumption of such oils over a long time could result in a gradual depletion—and eventual deficiency—of vitamin E.

It is difficult to obtain protective levels of vitamin E from diet alone. Recognized food sources of vitamin E include oils, nuts, seeds, and green leafy vegetables; however, dietary sources high in vitamin E are often high in fat. To get 100 IU daily a person would have to consume seven cups of peanuts, two cups of corn oil, or nineteen cups of spinach. Protective levels are also substantially higher than the current recommended dietary allowance (RDA) for vitamin E, which is only 10 mg (15 IU) for men and 8 mg (12 IU) for women.

HOW MUCH SUPPLEMENTAL VITAMIN E WILL PROTECT YOUR HEART?

Harvard's Dr. Rimm says he takes 200 IU of vitamin E a day but notes that "we shouldn't expect a single entity to significantly lower our risk. You need a combination of low fat, high fiber, fruit-and-vegetable-rich diet, plus exercise. But the benefits of supplementing with vitamin E do outweigh the risks.

"I think the strongest evidence that it was vitamin E that had this effect is that we looked at every other nutrient. If people who take vitamins are simply healthier, than people who take other vitamin supplements should have a lower rate of heart disease as well. But after we adjusted for vitamin E intake, there just weren't any other vitamins that reduced the risk of heart disease," Dr. Rimm explains.[38]

Dr. William A. Pryor, a researcher at Louisiana State University, says, "It is necessary to take a supplement to obtain the protective levels indicated by the scientific research."[39]

Dr. Jialal, the busy Southwestern Medical Center vitamin E researcher, has found that you need at least 400 IU of vitamin E each day to keep LDL from the hazardous oxidation. He recommends 200 IU twice a day.

A November 1996 survey of doctors attending the American Heart Association's annual conference found that 57 percent of the physicians had recommended antioxidant vitamins including vitamin E to patients at risk for heart disease, and 40 percent of the doctors took antioxidant supplements themselves.

There is certainly enough evidence to indicate that vitamin E is vital to the blood vessels and to the heart. Whether we all get sufficient vitamin E for this purpose or whether the low-cholesterol, polyunsaturated diet may deplete the body of the vital vitamin is still open to question. Certainly it deserves further scientific attention.

The Shute brothers, mentioned at the beginning of this chapter, gave their patients a small orange pamphlet called the "A.B.C. of Vitamin E." The pamphlet says that "vitamin

E improves the ability of the body to utilize oxygen as no other physiological substance can" and that "it is relative insurance against blood clots, whether in the coronary artery, or the brain, or the leg. The use of vitamin E is simple, cheap, and safe. It never causes hemorrhage. Vitamin E opens up unused blood vessels to give you detours around blocks you have in your circulation....The dose of vitamin E must be tailored to each person's needs. Vitamin E is a preventative as well as a treatment. We believe everyone should take it on that account."

If something as harmless and inexpensive as vitamin E could reduce the toll from cardiovascular disease, it would be of great benefit. In the United States alone, an estimated 7.9 million Americans age fifteen and older have disabilities resulting from cardiovascular conditions. Heart disease is the number-one killer, taking as many lives each year as the next eight leading causes of death combined. About one-sixth of the people killed by cardiovascular disease are under the age of sixty-five.[40]

In the 1970s, the Shutes noted, "The dose [of vitamin E] that fits your needs may not be approximately the dose your brother or uncle needs, even if he has your type of disease and is your height and weight. The dose must be tailored to each person's needs."

That's still excellent advice!

5

VITAMIN E AND CANCER

Since the 1960s, scientists have believed that cancer develops in two steps:

Step One: Initiation. Some substances, such as tobacco smoke, serve as initiators that start but cannot finish the cancer-causing process without the help of promoters.

Step Two: Promotion. Most promoters cannot work in cells that have not been initiated. Interfering with promoters offers the best approach in our lifetime of reducing cancer incidence. This was demonstrated, for example, when the "promoter" estrogen supplementation given to post-menopausal women was found to cause cancer of the uterine lining. When the estrogen medication was curtailed, the cases of endometrial cancer in postmenopausal women dropped dramatically. Saccharin is another cancer promoter (although a weak one), hence the warning on the artificial sweetener's packaging.[1]

In most instances exposure to cancer-causing agents (carcinogens) takes place twenty to thirty years before a statistically significant increase in cancer can be detected. Only then can it be adduced that the increase in cancer may have been caused by exposure to specific cancer-causing agents.

Each of us is unique in the way our body processes chemicals, based on our age, sex, heredity, medical history, diet, and behavior. Epidemiologists estimate that approximately one-third of all cancer deaths can be attributed to diet.[2]

Since we are all exposed to cancer-causing agents in our food, air, home, and at work, many scientists believe the best hope for preventing the development of the disease is to have something protect us at the promotion stage.

Some eminent scientists believe that vitamin E protects the cell against cancer-inducing agents, particularly those in air pollution and food. Although the studies on cancer and vitamin E are not as far advanced as those concerning blood and cardiovascular disease, it is theorized that the vitamin may protect us against cancer by stimulating our immune systems and/or protecting the DNA, the genetic information in our cells.[3] When a virus, a chemical, or some other cancer-inducing agent damages the DNA and fouls up the genetic information, the cells become abnormal. Cancer is an abnormal growth of cells.

As far back as 1962, researchers found that when female mice received thirty to one hundred times the normal dietary intake of vitamin E and were injected just under the skin with a powerful cancer-causing agent, only half as many tumors appeared in the vitamin E group as in the controls. An additional experiment with male mice showed a 50 percent reduction in those fed the high-vitamin-E diet.[4] However, in another study, vitamin E did not suppress tumors in mice given another powerful cancer-causing agent by injection.[5]

There are a number of explanations of how vitamin E might protect against cancer. Just as you have read in earlier chapters, culprits that play a part in cell damage are free radicals, those products of our metabolism that act like loose cannons. Researchers speculate vitamin E has the ability to stabilize those loose cannons and keep them from damaging our DNA.

Dr. Robert E. Olson of St. Louis University, on the other hand, an authority on lipid biochemistry and physiology, startled his colleagues at a 1987 symposium by suggesting that vitamin E and other fat-soluble vitamins may be the handmaidens of the genes that regulate the making of the enzymes, the workhorses of the cell.[6]

Vitamin E can, according to Dr. Olson's hypothesis, repress the production of enzymes by the genes, while vitamins A, D, and K are promoters of enzyme manufacture. Dr. Olson believes that vitamin E deficiency removes the repression mechanism that normally keeps certain genes inactive. When these particular genes go awry, cancer may develop.

Another link between cancer and vitamin E may be in that vitamin E has been found by many scientists to "spare" vitamin A. Vitamin A is believed by a number of researchers to protect against intestinal cancer.

T. Keith Murray, Ph.D., of the Nutrition Division of the Canadian Food and Drug Directorate, revealed an unexplained and "shocking" incidence of probable vitamin A deficiency in his native land, one of the better-fed nations in the world. In a report made at the Western Hemisphere Nutrition Congress in Puerto Rico in August 1968, he said evidence was gathered in autopsies of one hundred persons ten years and older that showed they had seriously depleted stores of vitamin A. The liver is a storage depot for vitamin A. More than 30 percent of the deceased had no more vitamin A in liver storage than is customarily found in newborn infants.

"Clearly, a high proportion of Canadians were in unsatisfactory vitamin A status at the time of death," Dr. Murray

said. "No clear pattern relating low stores to a particular disease has emerged, however, and we suspect that some environmental factors—drugs, pesticides, food additives,
etc.—may be reducing the utilization or increasing the
metabolism of vitamin A."

Could lack of vitamin E—and consequent failure to protect stores of vitamin A—be this factor?

Vitamin A and vitamin E work together. In fact, twenty-
five years after the Canadian study was presented, Japanese
researchers at the University of Tokushima reported that giving rats increased amounts of vitamin E and A activated the
function of lung cells that protect us against bacteria and foreign substances. The researchers surmised that these defensive cells are probably stimulated by the fat-soluble vitamins
A and E coming into the lung via the intestines. Thus, they
said they believe vitamin E will be especially important in
preventing lung infections and cancer.[7]

LUNG CANCER, AIR POLLUTION, AND VITAMIN E

Can vitamin E protect the lungs against air pollution, which
might lead to cancer?

Ozone is a variant of oxygen classed as a photochemical
because it is created by the action of sunlight. Ozone is a powerful oxidizing agent. Most news stories have warned of a
hazardous lack of ozone, of holes in the "ozone layer," allow-
ing penetration by deadly levels of ultraviolet. Here on earth,
however, ozone poses a peril because it is an air pollutant.
This intensely irritating gas can have devastating effects on
respiration, perpetrating lung damage similar to that caused
by smoking.[8]

In a 1969 report by the American Chemical Society entitled "Clean Our Environment," it was pointed out that rats exposed to one part per million of ozone-contaminated air eight hours daily for about a year had severe lung damage, and that healthy humans exposed to two parts per million of ozone for one hour had serious interference with their lung function.

Dr. Aloys L. Tappel, University of California professor of food science and technology, reported in May 1971 that rats fed vitamin E deficient diets were more adversely affected by ozone air pollution than rats fed vitamin E supplemented diets.

"The results show the increased sensitivity to ozone of the animals fed lower levels of vitamin E," Dr. Tappel said. "Death from acute lung edema [accumulation of an excessive amount of fluid] caused by ozone correlated with the lack of vitamin E in the diet. This evidence, together with the background knowledge of vitamin E function, strongly supports the current recommendation of the Food and Nutrition Board for adequate daily intake of vitamin E, particularly among those persons exposed to smog."

Even then, fats made rancid by oxygen were thought to be the cause of ozone's cancer-causing effects. But only recently have human studies really begun to add great weight to the earlier observations about antioxidant vitamin E being protective against cancer.

More than twenty-five years after his report on ozone and vitamin E, Dr. Tappel is still proving that vitamin E in the diet and other antioxidants protect livers, kidneys, and other tissues from oxygen damage.[9]

DIET, VITAMIN E, AND COLON CANCER

One of the first to associate our modern diet and cancer was Dr. Denis P. Burkitt of London, whose epidemiological studies reported a link between the concentrated, low-residue, refined diets of Americans and other Westerners with the great prevalence of rectal and colon cancer. In countries with a high-residue, bulky, unrefined diet, there is a low incidence of this type of cancer. Dr. Burkitt believed that high-residue diets are eliminated faster than low-residue, refined diets, and the action on the intestines of chemical and bacterial contaminants in the waste material may be the cause of the high incidence of bowel cancer. Bulky, high-residue diets are rich in vitamin E.

Although controlled human studies on the antioxidants and cancer are limited, the majority of epidemiological data suggest that vitamin E and the other antioxidants may decrease cancer incidence. In several studies, subjects with the highest serum concentration of vitamin E and other antioxidants had a lower subsequent risk of certain cancers than did subjects with lower serum antioxidant concentrations.

Can vitamin E also thwart or at least delay the onset of colon cancer, the second leading cause of cancer death in the United States?

Dr. Robert M. Bostick, of the University of Minnesota, and his colleagues wanted to find out. They investigated whether large amounts of antioxidants including vitamin E had an impact on the development of colon cancer among thirty-five thousand women, aged fifty-five to sixty-nine. The scientists reviewed the subjects' dietary questionnaires, which provided information on food intake, and vitamin and mineral use. In a retrospective review of the participants' health records, they cited 212 cases of colon cancer that had developed during the five-year follow-up period. The researchers discovered those who had developed the disease reported significantly lower intakes of vitamin E (dietary and supplemental vitamin E combined) than women who remained free of the disease.[10]

"After adjusting for age, we found a strong link between vitamin E and the incidence of colon cancer," says Dr. Bostick. "Most notably, we saw a big jump in the *decrease* of colon cancer at a daily intake of just thirty IUs. Further, the risk decreased progressively as the amount of vitamin E intake increased." The effects were most apparent in women younger than sixty-five.

Dr. Bostick agreed with the theories that vitamin E may protect against free radical damage and may increase immunity, but he believes it also protects against nitrosamines.

VITAMIN E AND NITROSAMINES

What are nitrosamines and why should we care?

Nitrosamines are highly potent cancer-causing agents. They are derived from nitrates and nitrites in our food and water combining with natural food and stomach chemicals called amines.

Our major intake of nitrates in foodstuffs comes from vegetables, water supplies, or from nitrates as additives in meat-curing.[11]

Potassium nitrate, also known as saltpeter and niter, and *sodium nitrate,* also called Chile saltpeter, are used as color fixatives in the more than $125-billion-a-year cured-meat business.

Nitrates change into nitrites on exposure to air.

The nitrites are also food additives. *Potassium nitrite* is used as a color fixative in cured meats. *Sodium nitrite* has the peculiar ability to react chemically with the myoglobin molecule and impart red-bloodedness to processed meats, to convey tanginess to the palate, and to resist the growth of *Clostridium botulinum* spores. It is used as a color fixative in cured meats, bacon, bologna, frankfurters, deviled ham, meat spread, potted meats, spiced ham, Vienna sausages, smoke-cured tuna fish products, and in smoke-cured shad and salmon.

Nitrites, as pointed out, combine with natural stomach and food chemicals (secondary amines) to create nitrosamines, among the most powerful cancer-causing agents known.

Researchers at Michael Reese Medical Center linked infinitesimal amounts of nitrite to cancer in young laboratory mice, especially in the liver and lungs. Dr. Koshlya Rijhsinghani and her colleagues gave single doses (either 0.315 or 0.625 micrograms) of nitrosamine for each gram of the animal's weight. This method differs from the way other researchers have induced cancer in mice with nitrosamines by repeated small doses or single large doses. Nitrosamines also produce cancer in hamsters similar to pancreatic cancers in humans.[12]

The U.S. Department of Agriculture, which has jurisdiction over processed meats, and the FDA, which has jurisdiction over processed poultry, asked manufacturers to show that the use of nitrites was safe and that nitrosamines were not formed in the products as preliminary tests had shown in bacon. Processors claimed there was no chemical substitute for nitrite. They said alternative processing methods could be used, but the products would not look or taste the same.

Baby-food manufacturers voluntarily removed nitrites from baby foods in the early seventies.

The FDA found that adding the antioxidant vitamin C to processed meats prevents or at least retards the formation of nitrosamines. In May 1978, the USDA announced plans to require bacon manufacturers to reduce their use of nitrite from 150 to 120 ppm and to use preservatives that retard nitrosamine formation. Processors would have been required to keep nitrosamine levels to 10 ppm under the interim plan. But in August 1978 a new concern about nitrite was raised. The USDA and the FDA issued a joint announcement that the substance had been directly linked to cancer by a Massachusetts Institute of Technology study. That work was later disputed. In 1982, amyl and butyl nitrites used by homosexual men were linked to Kaposi's sarcoma and other abnormalities of the immune system.

In 1980, the FDA revoked its proposed phaseout because manufacturers said there was no adequate substitute for nitrites. In 1977, Germany banned nitrites and nitrates except in certain species of fish. However, a Committee on Nitrite and Alternative Curing Agents in Food, formed by the National Research Council in the United States, concluded that no single agent or process could replace nitrite completely: "Several chemical and physical treatments appear to be comparable in inhibiting outgrowth of *Clostridium botulinum* spores in types of meat products, but none confers the color and flavor that consumers have come to expect in nitrite-cured meats."

To reduce nitrosamines in bacon, the U.S. Department of Agriculture requires meatpackers to add sodium ascorbate or sodium erythrobate (vitamin Cs) to the curing brine. This offers only a partial barrier because ascorbate is soluble in water and its activity in fat is limited. Vitamin E, however, inhibits nitrosation in fatty tissues. The committee suggested that both C and E be added to provide more complete protection.

Why not ban nitrites from food?

The advocates of such changes point out nitrites as an example of risk and benefit. Nitrites combine with natural stomach chemicals to cause nitrosamines, powerful cancer-causing agents, but nitrites also prevent botulism, a potentially fatal illness caused by contaminated food. Since, advocates claim, there is no good substitute for nitrites, their benefits outweigh their risks. Until the all-purpose agent comes along or until consumer preferences change, the best compromise will probably be continued use of nitrite in conventional amounts with vitamins C and E added to block formation of nitrosamines, or the use of smaller amounts of nitrite in combination with biological acidification, irradiation, or the chemicals potassium sorbate, sodium hypophosphite, or fumarate esters, the committee said.

Vitamin E inhibits the conversion of nitrites to nitrosamine in the stomach.[13] In animal and cell-culture studies, vitamins E and C, acting as scavengers of nitrite compounds, prevented the formation of cancer-promoting nitrosamines.[14]

Researchers at the University of Arizona's Health Sciences Center found, for example, that vitamin E protected mice against esophageal cancers. (The esophagus is that portion of the digestive canal between the throat and stomach.) The mice were exposed to a potent carcinogen, a nitrosamine (N-nitrosomethylbenzylamine [NMBza]). Some of the mice were then infected with a virus that lowered their immunity. Some of the animals were then fed diets containing 30 IU of vitamin E. The mice that were fed vitamin E had decreased size and frequency of esophageal tumors in both the immunocompromised and nonimmunocompromised mice. The results suggest that vitamin E plays an antioxidant function that retards the incidence of esophageal cancers in both immunocompromised and nonimmunocompromised animals.[15]

So, if you must eat nitrite-laced meat or other food, drink something high in vitamin C—for example, orange juice, grapefruit juice, cranberry juice—or eat lettuce.[16] Evidence for this advice was gathered in American-financed studies in China.

CHINA STUDIES

Nitrosamines were also among the suspects in the high rate of human esophageal cancers in Linxian, China. There, cancers of this connector between the throat and stomach are one hundred times higher than in the United States.

This disparity in cancer rates initially drew attention from epidemiologists looking to decipher the causal factor or factors for these cancers. In the United States, tobacco and alcohol use are risk factors for the disease, but the Linxian population uses little tobacco or alcohol. Possible factors investigated besides nitrosamines were mycotoxins (substances produced by fungi in stored foods), silica (microscopic bits of hard minerals) in the grain, and a tendency to gulp down scalding-hot tea, but no clear culprit emerged.

Because studies throughout the world had shown that people who eat more fresh fruits and vegetables had a lower risk of cancer, especially the esophageal and stomach cancers prevalent in Linxian, a nutritional intervention study was initiated. The overall diet of the Linxian population is low in fruits, meats, and other animal products, and blood levels of micronutrients such as vitamins A, B, C, and E are low by Western standards.

"If vitamins work to help prevent cancer, then they were going to work in this population, where the people have had a consistently poor intake of several vitamins and minerals, and the cancers we were trying to prevent are known to be diet-related," said William Blot, Ph.D., of the Division of Cancer Etiology, National Cancer Institute.[17]

To test the largest number of potentially preventative vitamins and minerals, the researchers combined compounds that had similar or synergistic qualities at levels one to two times the U.S. recommended daily allowances. The compounds, called factors, were:

Factor A. Retinol, a form of vitamin A, (5,000 IU) plus zinc (as 22.5 mg of zinc oxide), which enhances the delivery of retinol to tissues.

Factor B. Riboflavin (3.2 mg) and niacin (40 mg), two B vitamins that are lacking in the local diet in the county.

Factor C. Vitamin C (as 120 mg of ascorbic acid) and molybdenum (as 30 mcg of molybdenum yeast complex), which may inhibit the formation and activity of nitrosamines, cancer-causing compounds found in some preserved foods.

Factor D. The antioxidants beta-carotene (15 mg) and vitamin E (as 30 mg of alpha tocopherol) with selenium (as 50 mcg of selenium yeast) were studied as factor D. Antioxidants are compounds that pair with carcinogens to prevent them from damaging DNA.

Beginning in March 1986, the participants in the General Population Trial in China were randomly assigned to take one or more factors (A and B, or A and C, or B and D, etc.), so that half of the people would be taking each factor. This design permitted analysis of the benefits of each group of nutrients. The participants took the supplements for five and a quarter years, until May 1991. After five years of supplementation, the group receiving beta-carotene, vitamin E, and selenium showed significant benefits, with the effects beginning to appear less than two years into the trial. The biggest benefit was the reduction in the cancer death rate, the principal cause of death in Linxian. Heart disease is uncommon in this region.

Of the 792 cancer deaths that occurred in the participants during the General Population Trial, 691 were from cancer of the esophagus or stomach, 32 from lung cancer, 28 from liver cancer, and less than 10 cases each from other types of cancers. For the participants taking the antioxidants (factor D), the number of deaths from esophageal cancer was reduced about 4 percent and deaths from stomach cancer were reduced 21 percent. Factor D, of course, included vitamin E and beta-carotene, another antioxidant. The number of cases of cancer diagnosed during that time (incidence) also decreased due to factor D. Seven percent fewer cancers were diagnosed overall—6 percent fewer esophageal and gastric cancers, and 12 percent fewer other cancers.

Strokes were the other major cause of death, accounting for 228 deaths, or 25 percent of total deaths. Deaths from stroke were reduced 10 percent in the group taking factor D.

FINNISH STUDY ON CANCER

The association between serum vitamin E levels and the subsequent incidence of cancer was also investigated in Finland, and the results were published in the *American Journal of Epidemiology*.[18] This longitudinal study involved 21,172 men initially aged fifteen to ninety-nine in six geographic areas of the country. The baseline examination was conducted in 1968 to 1972, and during the follow-up of six to ten years, 453 cancers were diagnosed. The vitamin E in the blood was measured from stored serum samples from these men and from 841 male controls, matched to municipality and age, who did not develop cancer during the follow-up. The mean levels of serum alpha tocopherol among the cancer cases and controls were 8.02 and 8.28 mg/l, respectively. A high serum vitamin E level was associated with a reduced risk of cancer. The association was strongest for the combined group of cancers unrelated to smoking and varied between groups of the study population as well as between different cancers. The association persisted when adjusted for serum cholesterol and other confounding factors. These findings agree with the hypothesis that high vitamin E intake protects against cancer, the researchers concluded.

ORAL CANCER AND VITAMIN E

New evidence suggests that the antioxidant properties of vitamin E may cut—in half—the risk of oral and throat cancers. The use of vitamin and mineral supplements was assessed in a population-based, case-control study of oral and throat cancer, conducted during 1984 to 1985 in four areas of the United States. There was no association with intake of multivitamin products, but users of the individual antioxidant vitamins including vitamins E, A, B, and C were at lower risk after controlling for the effects of tobacco. After further adjustment for use of other supplements, vitamin E was the only supplement that remained associated with significantly reduced cancer risk. Dr. G. Gridley and his colleagues at the National Cancer Institute's division of Cancer Etiology wrote in the *American Journal of Epidemiology* in 1992 that to the authors' knowledge, theirs was the first epidemiologic study to show a reduced oral cancer risk with vitamin E use. Although it is not clear that the lower risk among consumers of vitamin E supplements is due to the vitamin per se, the findings are consistent with experimental evidence and should prompt further research on the role of vitamin E and other micronutrients as inhibitors of oral and throat cancer.[19]

Three years earlier, the same group reported in the *Journal of the National Cancer Institute* that a population-based, case-control study of oral and pharyngeal cancer conducted in four areas of the United States showed that fruit was helpful in preventing oral and pharyngeal cancer. Individuals in the highest quartile of fruit intake had about half the risk of those in the lowest quartile. "Vitamin E carotene or fiber in fruit did not appear to account completely for this relationship," they reported, "since these nutrients in vegetables did not provide similar protection. This finding suggests the influence of other constituents in fruits, although it is possible that cooking vegetables may have a nutrient-diminishing effect. Dietary intake of other nutrients, such as the B vitamins, vitamin E, folate, and iron showed no consistent relationship to the risk of oral and pharyngeal cancer."[20]

PARTNERSHIP—SELENIUM AND VITAMIN E

Selenium, a trace metal that has been identified as a wind-blown contaminant, is believed to be released when fossil fuels are burned. Selenium, more than any other trace metal, illustrates the narrow line between vital and poisonous. In minute amounts it is essential to animal life, but it is more toxic than arsenic and mercury, and it is less abundant in the earth's crust than gold. It is essential to animal growth, but too much of it causes hooves to break off and hair to fall out; too little results in white muscle disease in calves and lambs. But selenium may help protect against cancers of the lung, colon, rectum, and prostate.

In 1957, a relationship was discovered between selenium and the antioxidant vitamin E. The vitamin lessened the amount of selenium required to prevent a common blood disorder in chicks, liver destruction in rats, the destruction of the gizzard and heart in turkeys, and the deterioration of muscles in lambs and calves.

The specific biochemical role of selenium in the prevention of these ailments and the mechanism of the interrelationship between vitamin E and selenium are not known. Minute amounts of selenium, it has been proven, can prevent some vitamin E deficiency diseases. Although no one knows for sure, some scientists believe that selenium aids the absorption of vitamin E into fat.

As far back as 1970, Dr. Raymond J. Shamburger of the Department of Clinical Pathology of the Cleveland Clinic Foundation in Ohio reported in the *Journal of the National Cancer Institute* that he found both vitamin E and selenium, given separately, reduce the number of animals that developed cancer when injected with a powerful cancer-inducing chemical. Yet when another antioxidant was substituted for vitamin E, it did not protect against cancer.

Daily supplementation with vitamins C and E resulted in a decrease in the average concentration of oxidized fat in the blood in a study of elderly people in Poland. In an evaluation of the effects of vitamin E and selenium supplementation on the mental well-being of nursing-home patients in Finland, a noted improvement in general condition was observed after only two months. In another Finnish study, oxidized fat in blood serum was initially higher in the elderly people but decreased to the same amount as that in young control subjects after three months of supplementation with vitamins C, E, and B$_6$, beta-carotene, zinc, and selenium.[21]

In a recent study while researchers were attempting to determine whether selenium could prevent certain types of skin cancer, they found some startling results. In a study of 1,312 patients with previous skin cancers, 200 mcg of the trace element were taken each day for an average of 4.5 years. The subjects were recruited from an area of the United States low in selenium in the soil.[22]

The researchers found the trace metal did not prevent recurrence of skin cancer. Midway through the study, however, the authors decided to also evaluate the effect of selenium for preventing other types of cancers and for reducing cancer mortality. Lo and behold, the selenium group had a 37 percent reduction in cancer incidence compared to the control group, and a 50 percent reduction in cancer mortality.

Of the nearly two hundred new cases of cancer diagnosed, the selenium group had 63 percent fewer prostate cancers, 59 percent fewer colorectal cancers, and 46 percent fewer lung cancers than the placebo group.

In a related editorial in the same issue of *Journal of the American Medical Association,* Dr. Graham A. Colditz, of Brigham and Women's Hospital and Harvard Medical School, Boston, Massachusetts, sounded a strong note of caution about the study and its findings. He wrote, "This promising set of results...require coordination in further randomized trials designed to test the effect of selenium supplementation on cancer incidence and mortality....For now it is premature to change individual behavior, to market specific selenium supplements, or to make public health recommendations based on the results of this one randomized trial."

He continued, "As we await the results of further prevention research, known lifestyle changes that can reduce cancer risks (such as smoking cessation, consuming adequate amounts of fruits and vegetables each day, reducing intake of animal fat, and increasing physical activity) should be implemented."

It is believed that selenium may protect against heart damage. At the same time, it is believed that in larger amounts it may cause heart damage and blood pressure changes.

Vitamin E protects cell membranes, works in blood, protects vitamin A and selenium. It has been theorized that we need 50 to 200 mcg of selenium to protect us from smog and smoke and to stave off cancer.

Deliberate addition of selenium to foods or animal feeds is prohibited in the United States. The federal tolerance level of selenium in drinking water is 0.01 parts per million, but there is no federal tolerance level for it in foods at this time. Selenium can be found in organ meats, seafood, meats, cereals and grains, egg yolks, mushrooms, onions, garlic.

6

VITAMIN E AND MUSCLE POWER

Coaches swear by it. Joggers gulp it down before running. Trainers give it to racehorses. All maintain that vitamin E increases muscle performance. What part does vitamin E play in muscle, a substance described by one researcher as "the most remarkable stuff in nature's curiosity shop"?

From the winking of an eye to the lifting of a heavy carton, we all take for granted those bundles of fibers. Yet the simple act of walking across the room or picking up an object dwarfs in complexity the workings of the most complicated man-made computer. In fact, the operations of the muscles are so complicated that science still does not fully understand them. They do know that muscle makes up 40 percent of our total weight, and that there are two main types of muscle, *voluntary* and *involuntary*.

The voluntary muscles, sometimes called skeletal muscles, are used to walk, run, lift heavy loads, support weight on our backs, or turn our heads. Their function is the movement and support of our skeletons. There are about 620 voluntary muscles, each with its own name, nerve supply, function, and points of origin and insertion. They are called striated muscle because, as can be seen under the microscope, they have

stripes. In healthy people, the voluntary muscles will shorten
or contract on demand.

To every rule there is an exception, and the heart muscle is
one. Under the microscope it is striated, but (except for a few
people such as yogis) we can't control its beating. It is therefore called an involuntary striated muscle.

Smooth muscle fibers, on the other hand, are shorter in
length and of smaller diameter than striated muscle. These
fibers are arranged in sheets rather than bundles. Several
sheets may lie on top of each other, but within each sheet all
the fibers run in the same direction. The sheets are arranged
so that the direction of fibers in one sheet is different from
those on either side. The smooth muscles make up the muscular layers of the intestines, blood vessels, and bladder. We
have no conscious control over them.

The expression "muscles of iron" is frequently used. Yet
the working or contractile element in the muscle is only jelly.
And how this jelly contracts instantaneously to lift as much as
a thousand times its own weight is a miracle—and a mys-
tery—of human machinery. An elaborate series of chemical
and electrical actions requiring days to duplicate in a laboratory takes place instantly when we contract a muscle in such
simple actions as pursing our lips for a kiss or throwing a ball.

Performance of strenuous physical activity can increase
oxygen consumption by ten- to fifteenfold over rest to meet
energy demands. Again, the elevated oxygen consumption,
particularly by the skeletal muscles, produces an "oxidative
stress" that leads to the generation of free radicals and subse-
quently deposits of rancid fat (lipid peroxidation).[1]

Many metabolic changes occur in heavily exercised muscles, leading to alteration in the relative concentrations of fat
and water. A German study shows that in humans vitamin E

prevents exercise-induced DNA damage and indicates that DNA breakage occurs in white blood cells after exhaustive exercise as a consequence of oxidative stress.[2]

Researchers affiliated with the U.S. Department of Agriculture have shown that vitamin E taken before exercise can minimize muscle damage and reduce inflammation and soreness that so often follows strenuous exercise.[3]

Dr. S. N. Meydani and colleagues at the Antioxidant Research Laboratory and Human Physiology at the USDA Human Nutrition Research Center on Aging at Tufts University, Boston, studied the protective effect of vitamin E supplementation on exercise-induced oxidative damage in twenty-one male volunteers.[4]

Nine young men aged twenty-two to twenty-nine and twelve older men fifty-four to seventy-four, who all were sedentary, participated in a double-blind (see glossary) protocol. They received either 800 IU vitamin E daily or a placebo. After forty-eight days, vitamin E supplementation significantly increased vitamin E levels in the blood and skeletal muscles. Subjects then performed a bout of eccentric exercise at 75 percent of their maximum heart rate by running down an inclined treadmill for forty-five minutes. Twelve days postexercise, all vitamin-E-supplemented subjects excreted less telltale substances signifying oxygen-produced cell damage than those who received only placebos. This benefit was noted in men over fifty-five as well as those in their twenties. The vitamin also reduced blood levels of two chemical messengers that promote inflammation, which should reduce postexercise inflammation and soreness.

Other researchers have found similar results with vitamin E and exercise.

Dr. Phyllis Clarkson, Department of Exercise Science,

University of Massachusetts, for example, examined indirect measurements of free radicals generated during exercise. One of these included pentane exhaled in the breath, which is a telltale sign of oxidized fat.[5] Healthy subjects who received 1,200 IU/day of a tocopherol for two weeks had significantly lower pentane production while resting and exercising than nonsupplemented controls.

In another study, pentane production more than doubled in a group of high-altitude mountain climbers. When the climbers took 400 mg of a tocopherol per day, they showed no significant elevation in pentane exhalation.[6] Thus under some circumstances, vitamin E may protect muscles from exercise-induced free radical injury.[7]

Physical training has been shown to result in an augmented antioxidant system and a reduction in rancid fat (lipid peroxidation), according to Dr. Clarkson. The "weekend athletes" may not have the augmented antioxidant defense system produced through continued training, she says. This may make them more susceptible to oxidative stress.

Patients with coronary heart disease can also better tolerate exercise if supplemented with vitamin E, according to Russian researchers.[8] And there was also a report that vitamin E can help prevent damage to the heart muscle during exercise, at least in rats.[9]

These findings about vitamin E and exercise support the recommendation of Dr. Lester Packer that people with active lifestyles should consider increasing daily dietary vitamin E intake, because endurance training in animal studies has demonstrated depletion of body vitamin E reserves when a normal diet is consumed.[10]

Researchers have also investigated the effects of vitamin E

supplementation on athletic performance. Racehorses and rats have been reported to race better with their muscles protected by vitamin E.[11] In two studies, however, vitamin-E-supplemented, trained swimmers did not show a difference in swimming speed compared with swimmers on a placebo diet.[12]

William Evans, Ph.D., and his colleagues at the University of Pennsylvania's Center for Sports Medicine studied the effects of vitamin E on muscle during weight lifting. They typically accepted subjects from fifty-five to eighty years old in their exercise lab at the university. They also conducted studies in nursing homes, with no age limit on participants.[13]

Dr. Evans points out that "any exercise to which you are unaccustomed can cause mechanical damage including destruction of muscle proteins. What we were interested in was the influence of vitamin E on the repair of muscle. There are certain aspects of the immune system that are associated with the repair of muscle. When a muscle is damaged, immune cells take action, invade the muscle, and take away damaged tissue. They help repair and make the muscle stronger. We found vitamin E had little effect on young people whose immune system is strong. However, in people over fifty years, vitamin E did have a significant benefit for muscle repair."[14]

Dr. Evans and his group are now working to determine the effects of exercise on dietary protein requirements and the influence of nutrition on muscle. He said they have found strength training reduces the need for protein. The more you exercise with weights, the more you retain of the protein. He said they have had good results with weight lifting in persons with wasting diseases and chronic kidney failure.

He says of exercise and vitamin E that there is "good

strong evidence that vitamin E has a lot of positive effects. In our study, we gave subjects eight hundred IU of vitamin E twice a day, which is probably excessive. We think that two hundred to four hundred IU per day is appropriate. You cannot get that much in the diet."

He said that vitamin E will not increase your athletic performance, but there is good evidence that vitamin E may enhance insulin action in diabetes. Exercise does that, too, so there may be a positive interaction for those with diabetes who exercise. Dr. Evans takes 200 IU of vitamin E a day.

The current conclusion from studies concerning vitamin E and exercise is that the vitamin helps to prevent damage to the muscles during exercise. This applies to weekend athletes as well as those performing regular heavy exercise.[15, 16] Researchers from Ireland, Italy, and Canada have reported protective benefit in their studies with vitamin E and exercise.[17]

Vitamin E supplementation of athletes has produced equivocal effects on performance, as noted above. The current consensus, based on well-controlled research, is that vitamin E supplementation does not improve athletic performance. However, it may play an important role in preventing exercise-induced muscle injury, and this may indirectly help performance, especially in marathon-type exercise.

In exercise-exhausted animals, free-radical concentrations are increased two- to threefold in muscle and the liver and accelerated oxidized-fat deposits and muscle-fiber damage have been observed.[18] More rapid depletion of vitamin E from liver and muscle have been observed in rats undergoing endurance training than in sedentary controls at similar vitamin E intakes. The fact that the primarily antioxidant vitamin E is consumed by body tissues during increased physical exercise, suggests that an increased vitamin E requirement during endurance training would be beneficial. In a study in human subjects, daily supplementation with 1,200 IU of vitamin E for two weeks significantly reduced the increased pentane production documented in strenuous physical exercise.[19] Pentane is a signal that free radicals are at work oxidizing fats.

A number of scientists suggest that vitamin E and C are protective but best obtained from fruits and vegetables rather than supplements.[20]

And finally, some say vitamin E may or may not protect your muscles somewhat during exercise, but in any case, it is not harmful.[21]

If you want to *jump* to a conclusion, you may as well take a vitamin E tablet or eat a lot of wheat germ before you do it.

AVOIDING LEG CRAMPS

Those joggers, swimmers, racers, and other athletes who maintain vitamin E helps them perform better do have some clinicians who believe they may know why. Doctors at the University of East Carolina School of Medicine report vitamin E can help counteract leg cramps that commonly bother people, especially athletes and the elderly. The diagnosis of cause may be heat, electrolyte disturbance, or most commonly "unknown."[22]

Treatments include stretching, quinine sulfate, and/or vitamin E.

Dr. S. J. Ayres and Dr. R. Mihan of the University of California at Los Angeles conducted studies in the 1970s with vitamin E for the treatment of leg cramps. They had given their first 102 cases an average of 300 to 400 IU (and occasionally 800 IU) of alpha tocopherol daily. They reported good results in *California Medicine*.[23]

"This series," they wrote, "includes six patients with restless legs, three with nocturnal rectal cramps, and one young athlete training for the Olympics who had severe cramps following strenuous exercise including long distance running, swimming, and weight lifting. All of these patients received prompt and gratifying relief from the oral administration of vitamin E."

Dr. Robert F. Cathcart III, a San Mateo, California, orthopedist, soon after decided to treat one hundred patients complaining of leg cramps with 300 IU of vitamin E daily. He reported in the *Journal of the American Medical Association* that the supplement was almost universally effective. He noted, however, that patients who reduced the dosage to 100 IU daily often found it inadequate.[24]

Since leg cramps can be the result of many physical conditions, it is best to check with your physician before trying to combat the discomfort with vitamin E.

WHAT ABOUT THOSE WITH SERIOUS MUSCLE PROBLEMS?

More than 5 million Americans have conditions that limit their ability to perform muscular work. Vitamin E deficiency has been found to develop in humans with such conditions as cystic fibrosis, celiac disease, sprue, blockage of the bile duct, biliary cirrhosis, and chronic pancreatitis, all of which produce a fat-absorption problem. Remember that most vitamin E is stored in fat.

The muscular dystrophies encompass a group of degenerative diseases of the voluntary or skeletal muscles, characterized by primary pathology in the muscle, not directly in the nervous system. Progression is rapid in some types and slow in others. As yet, no treatment can stop the relentless progression nor correct the underlying pathology in humans. But muscular dystrophy can be cured in animals!

One of the most common results of vitamin E deficiency in animals, including the rhesus monkey, is an acute and degenerative change in the skeletal muscles and, in some instances, the heart muscle—muscular dystrophy.

Dr. Max Horwitt, a pioneer in the metabolism of vitamin E in humans, pointed out in a paper published more than thirty-five years ago that the rabbit is a favorite experimental animal for the study of vitamin E deficiency because of the relative ease with which muscular dystrophy can be produced in it by withholding vitamin E.

"However, as far as is known," Dr. Horwitt wrote, "no one has correlated this ease of producing nutritional dystrophy in this animal with the fact that the deposits of fat in a rabbit— and presumably of its young—has a very high concentration of linolenic acid and other polyunsaturated fatty acids. Considering the leafy composition of the diets of most rabbits, it is possible that the ease with which vitamin E deficiency can be induced in rabbits is more a function of the rabbits' dietary history than a species difference."

Dr. Horwitt pointed out that muscle tissue rapidly accumulates polyunsaturated fats. He theorizes that the specific pathology obtained in a vitamin E deficient animal may depend not only upon an imbalance within a given tissue, but possibly also upon the fact that, after a muscle or nerve cell has lost its reserve of vitamin E, the transport of a toxic, oxidized product from a distant area of the body may trigger pathology such as muscular dystrophy.

Dr. Henry J. Binder of Yale, writing in the *New England Journal of Medicine,* December 9, 1965, pointed out that "muscular dystrophy is not usually found in persons deficient in tocopherol, nor is muscular dystrophy improved in any way by tocopherol therapy."

However, he said he found in humans classic signs of vitamin E deficiency as seen in animals—muscle weakness, ceroid (oxidized fat) deposits, and an increased excretion of creatine in the urine (a harbinger of muscular dystrophy), as well as increased red blood cell fragility. The deficiency did not show up for at least nine months after the onset of malabsorption (of fat) and sometimes not until eighteen to sixty months had elapsed.

Dr. Binder did find focal necrosis (dead spots) in skeletal muscles in a few patients with vitamin E deficiency, and in a case reported in the *New England Journal of Medicine,* there was a "strikingly similar" change between the muscles of the patient and those of tocopherol-deficient rabbits with muscular dystrophy. He reasoned that the pathological picture of muscle metabolism in vitamin E deficient patients suffering from fat malabsorption and in animals suffering from muscular dystrophy may mean that the characteristic muscle weakness that occurs in fat-malabsorption conditions such as sprue may be due to the lack of vitamin E in the body.

Dr. Binder said that in one case, ceroid (a brown pigment caused by changes in body fat) was found at autopsy in every smooth-muscle structure examined, including the heart muscle. He also pointed out that such ceroid deposits have been found in the muscle of every child over the age of five years dying of cystic fibrosis, an inherited disease of the exocrine glands, which pour secretions out of the body rather than into the blood. Cystic fibrotic children also cannot utilize fat properly.

One of the pioneers in vitamin E clinical research, Dr. Ade T. Milhorat, professor of clinical medicine at Cornell University Medical School and chairman of the Medical Board of the Muscular Dystrophy Associations of America, said in an interview in the 1970s, "Vitamin E deficiency presents an interesting pathological picture. The lesions in humans are quite similar to those induced by vitamin E deficiency in animals. We have used all sorts of vitamin E preparations, but none of them worked in human muscular dystrophy. I am reserved about saying that vitamin E will never work, until we know the full story of it."

Some scientists maintain that truly therapeutic doses of a strong vitamin E compound have not as yet been tried.

7

VITAMIN E AND YOUR LUNGS

Take a deep breath. Even the conservative American Lung Association says vitamin E may help your lungs!

At least 14.2 million Americans are estimated to suffer from chronic obstructive pulmonary disease, the fourth-ranking cause of death. And an estimated 11.7 million Americans suffer from asthma. Several recent studies published by the American Lung Association add to evidence that the antioxidant vitamins may have a beneficial effect on the lungs.

One study involved 2,633 adults in Nottingham, England, about half of whom had never smoked and 597 of whom were current smokers. All were questioned about their dietary intake of vitamin E and vitamin C, and their lung function was measured.

"We found that the higher their vitamin C intake, the better their pulmonary function," said Scott Weiss, M.D., a coauthor of the study and a volunteer spokesperson for the American Lung Association. Vitamin E alone did not appear to have an independent effect on lung function. But the researchers said it is not possible to distinguish clearly between the effects of the two vitamins, and they conclude it is likely that both vitamin C and vitamin E have a beneficial effect on lung function.[1]

WHAT ABOUT ASTHMA?

Asthma is a condition of difficult, labored, wheezy breathing. In the most common form, bronchial asthma, the arduous breathing is due to narrowing of the bronchial passages, which traps inhaled air and makes it hard to exhale. Allergy is often a cause.

Harvard researchers are following the health and diet habits of 77,866 women enrolled in the ongoing Nurses Health Study. In one aspect of the investigation, the scientists were trying to find links between diet and asthma.[2]

Initially, researchers found that the women who consumed the most vitamin E from foods (but not from supplements) were about half as likely to develop asthma compared to women who consumed the least vitamin E. But when they took into account that some women with asthma may avoid vitamin E rich nuts and peanut butter because they can bring on an allergic reaction, the researchers calculated that women who consumed the most vitamin E were 25 percent less likely to develop asthma compared with women who consumed the least.

The antioxidant vitamins may decrease airway inflammation and thereby decrease the severity of asthma or prevent asthma symptoms altogether in susceptible people, the researchers said.

British researchers who studied vitamin E and vitamin C in the diet reported in another study that the diets of Asian Indians living in Great Britain may protect them against asthma. The Indian diet is high in vegetables and fruits containing the antioxidant vitamins, and they have less asthma than other populations in Britain.[3]

The researchers asked parents of 539 Indian children and 308 white children ages eight to eleven in four schools in the English city of Leicester to complete questionnaires about their children's diets and other lifestyle factors, as well as their history of asthma and wheezing. The children were also given lung-function and allergy tests.

Indian children who ate the most Indian food were least likely to have abnormally sensitive airways, a sign of asthma. The study also found that the more Indian food they ate, the lower their risk of allergy.

This fits in with a study done in 1972 in which volunteers were injected with histamine, a substance released into the body when an allergic reaction occurs. Those who had been pretreated with vitamin E for five to seven days before showed far less swelling around the injection site than a control group that did not receive pretreatment with the vitamin.[4] This caused researchers to believe vitamin E has antihistamine properties.

KEEPING THE ELDERLY BREATHING

Aside from its possible beneficial effects in asthma, vitamin E has been reported to help preserve the lung function of elderly people. A study published by the American Lung Association involved 178 men and women age seventy and older. The results showed those who consumed the most vitamin E had significantly better lung function than those who consumed the least. No such effect was seen from vitamin C consumption, reported lead researcher Lindsey Dow, M.D., of Frenchay Hospital in Bristol, England. The elderly tend to have diets deficient in vitamins, Dr. Dow noted.[5]

Dr. Dow said that it is not known exactly how much vitamin E must be consumed to affect lung function. It is also not known whether vitamin E consumed in foods is more or less beneficial than vitamin E in pill form, she added.

SMOKERS, POLLUTION, AND LUNG FUNCTION

As pointed out in the chapter on vitamin E and cancer, the vitamin helps to protect the lung against air pollution. Ozone and nitrogen dioxide, present in high concentrations in polluted air, can initiate free-radical reactions that lead to lung injury. Cigarette smoke contains free radicals and compounds that generate free radicals and leads to a significant increase in the number of inflammatory cells in the lung, which are potent producers of free radicals. Vitamin E may be an important component of the lung's defense against free-radical-related injury. Research in rats showed a protective effect of vitamin E on the lungs of rats exposed to ozone or cigarette smoke.[6]

In a study of smokers, baseline breath-pentane excretion—a sign of free-radical oxidation—was significantly higher in smokers than nonsmokers, but breath pentane output was suppressed by daily supplementation with 800 IU vitamin E.[7] In another study, lower-respiratory-tract fluid of smokers was relatively deficient in vitamin E; vitamin E concentrations increased with daily intake of 2,400 IU vitamin E for three weeks but still remained much lower than baseline concentrations of nonsmokers. The researchers suggest that the vitamin E deficiency in young smokers may expose their lungs to increased free-radical damage.

Should you take supplemental vitamin E and vitamin C to protect your lungs?

"It's still too early to make recommendations, except for a

general recommendation that eating fresh fruits and vegetables, which are important sources of vitamins C and E, would clearly be beneficial," said Scott Weiss, M.D., a coauthor of several recent vitamin studies and a volunteer spokesperson for the American Lung Association.

"The most important thing you can do to prevent chronic obstructive pulmonary disease is not to smoke," said Dr. Weiss, associate professor of medicine at Harvard Medical School and Brigham and Women's Hospital in Boston, "but there may be some residual benefit from making sure you have an adequate intake of fresh fruits and vegetables."

8

VITAMIN E AND YOUR SKIN

The skin is our shield of armor, the mirror of our emotions, the largest organ of our body, and after the brain, the most complex. It can be afflicted by more than 2,100 diseases.

In an adult, the skin has an area of from 9,500 to 3,000 square inches and weighs about eight pounds. It has seventy-seven feet of nerves, nineteen feet of blood vessels, and 645 sweat glands per square inch. It protects the body against invasion by bacteria, the rays of the sun, and loss of moisture. It also protects from injury the more sensitive tissues within the body and serves as a sensitive organ of perception: it contains hundreds of pain, pressure, heat, and cold receptors.

The skin is generally soft and flexible and more elastic in younger people. It varies in thickness from one-fiftieth of an inch on the eyelids to as much as one-third of an inch on the palms and soles.

The skin is made up of three layers: the *epidermis,* the *dermis,* and the *subcutaneous* layer. The *subcutaneous layer* contains fat, blood vessels, and nerves. It links the *dermis* (middle layer) with tissues covering the muscles and bones. It also serves as the smooth and springy base of the skin.

Wrinkles appear as we grow older because the fatty tissue

is absorbed and the outer layers of the skin form uneven folds.

The top layer of the *epidermis,* the *stratum corneum* (sometimes called the *horny layer*), is made of scales that are actually dead skin cells. They gradually flake off or soak off when wet. The horny layer is constantly being replaced by cells pushed toward the surface as new cells are formed in the deeper layer of the epidermis.

More than any other organ, our skin is exposed to numerous environmental chemical and physical agents, such as ultraviolet light, causing oxidative stress. In the skin, this results in sunburn and dryness, and long term in wrinkles, thickening, "age spots," and even skin cancer.[1]

Sunlight is the most important cause of both prematurely aged skin and the most prevalent type of malignancy in humans, skin cancer.[2] As early as 1975 the Japanese performed experiments with mice in which alpha tocopheryl acetate ointment was applied to the skin prior to ultraviolet radiation and proved protective.

CAN VITAMIN E PROTECT OUR SKIN AGAINST THE RAVAGES OF THE SUN?

In several human studies, it has been shown that vitamin E in solution on the skin is protective against ultraviolet radiation. It diminishes oxidation of fat and the resulting tissue damage from the sun.[3]

Sunlight is made up of visible, infrared, and ultraviolet radiation. The ultraviolet radiation that reaches the earth's surface consists of ultraviolet A and ultraviolet B. Ultraviolet A rays have longer wavelengths than ultraviolet B and are of lower energy. Approximately a thousand times more ultraviolet A energy than ultraviolet B energy is needed to produce skin redness or sunburn. However, because the solar energy reaching the earth's surface contains ten to one hundred times more ultraviolet A than ultraviolet B, ultraviolet A can have significant effects on the body.

While the amount of ultraviolet B radiation reaching the earth's surface varies at different times of the day and during different seasons, the amount of ultraviolet A radiation is relatively constant. Ultraviolet B rays have long been known to be responsible for causing skin cancer and other skin damage, including sunburn. While ultraviolet B is the primary culprit in causing visible damage such as redness and sunburn, more and more evidence shows that ultraviolet A also has its dangers.[4]

Researchers at the North Carolina Biotechnology Center, Raleigh, North Carolina, found that a combination of both vitamins E and C form a good guard against UVB insult, the bulk of the protection attributable to vitamin E. However, vitamin C is significantly better than vitamin E at protecting against a UVA-mediated phototoxic insult, they reported.[5]

On the other hand, studies at the Cancer Prevention and Control Program, Arizona Cancer Center, Tucson, in mice showed that the application of the dl-alpha-tocopherol form of vitamin E to the skins of mice prevents skin cancer and the immunosuppression induced by all ultraviolet radiation. Arizona is a very sunny place. However, dl-alpha-tocopherol has limited stability at room temperature. Therefore, the Arizonans studied heat-stable esters of vitamin E—*alpha tocopheryl acetate* and *alpha tocopheryl succinate*—to prevent skin cancer due to ultraviolet radiation. (An ester is a compound formed from an alcohol and an acid by elimination of water.) They found that neither of the esters prevent skin cancer and may, in fact, have enhanced the process.[6]

"Considering that alpha tocopherol esters are included in

many skin lotions, cosmetics, and sunscreens, further studies are needed to determine the conditions under which topical alpha tocopheryl acetate and alpha tocopheryl succinate enhance photocarcinogenesis," the researchers said.

Research has shown, as pointed out above, that a close relationship exists between ultraviolet radiation, free radicals, oxidized fat, and tissue damage.

WHY VITAMIN E MAY WORK ON THE SKIN

Since vitamin E is essential to every tissue in the body and is known to have a profound effect on blood, blood vessels, and fat, it stands to reason that it is necessary for healthy skin.

Given the high vitamin E content of the pituitary and adrenal cortex, it is thought that the endocrine glands are centers of vitamin E metabolism. Since vitamin E is absorbed through the skin, it may have some beneficial effect as a hormone partner.

Electron microscopy examination of the skin has demonstrated that vitamin E ointment is a protectant for the skin and is capable of repairing epidermal cell damage caused by irritation. It also appears to have an anti-inflammatory effect.[7]

A marketing survey by Hoffmann–La Roche, one of the largest producers of vitamin E, found that 58 percent of the ingesters of vitamin E capsules also use the vitamin in creams, lotions, and even directly from soft gelatin capsules. The respondents said they believe vitamin E to be good for cuts, burns, age spots, dryness, and many other skin problems.[8] The scientific support for such claims is sparse. Nevertheless, users of creams, lotions, and salves containing vitamin E often swear by the result.

Vitamin E is used either alone or in combination with other materials for the treatment of chronic skin diseases. It has also been tried to aid wound healing, but studies thus far suggest that it has value only in reducing scarring, not in healing. This is probably due to its ability to inhibit excessive collagen formation at the wound site.[9] Collagen is an insoluble protein found in connective tissue.

Reduction of scarring was demonstrated as far back as 1972.[10] Anti-inflammatory actions were also reported in the early 1970s, and this was thought to be the result of suppression of histamine release.[11] Histamine is released into the body when an allergic reaction occurs. In the 1980s, studies confirmed vitamin E acetate at 5 percent and 100 percent as an anti-inflammatory agent on human skin.[12]

The effects of vitamin E may be limited to those of an antioxidant. Clinical evidence indicates that topical use of vitamin E may be helpful in the following conditions: acne, scar tissue, connective-tissue diseases, progressive scleroderma, scleroderma, dermatomyositis, and lupus erythematosus.

Dr. Samuel Ayres, Jr. and Dr. Richard Mihan of the University of California at Los Angeles reported in *California Medicine* they were using vitamin E to treat several rare and incurable skin diseases involving connective tissue. The diseases included scleroderma, a thickening of the skin caused by swelling and thickening of fibrous tissue, which leads to eventual atrophy of the skin and epidermolysis bullosa, a hereditary condition in which blisters are produced by slight rubbing of the skin because of degenerated elastic tissue. Dr. Ayres reported the results were "promising."

WHAT ABOUT VITAMIN E AND COSMETICS?

The benefits of vitamin E in topical products are based on the following:

It is readily absorbed through the skin.

It passes through the epidermis to the dermis.

It is absorbed through the hair follicles.

There is no absorption through the sebaceous glands or sweat glands.

There is little storage in the skin and limited data is available on the skin distribution of vitamin E after oral ingestion.

It blocks lipid peroxidation, which is involved in cell-membrane damage in tissues.

It enhances the performance of sun-care products by preventing UV rays from causing injury from peroxidation of the skin's fatty acids.

It moisturizes the skin from within.

It contributes to a smoother appearance of the skin.

It has been shown to reduce scarring from wounds.

It has anti-inflammatory properties.

It has been shown to help peripheral blood circulation.[13]

In 1991, Lester Packer, at the University of California at Berkeley, reported using several vitamin E creams on animal skin. His work shows as much as a fifteenfold increase in skin vitamin E levels after fifteen days of continual use. Further, he suggests an antioxidant protection using his newly developed ozone exposure assay.[14]

In human experiments to measure transepidermal water loss (TEWL), Italian researcher Dr. P. T. Pugliese tested a 5 percent concentration of vitamin E as a "moisturizer." Moisturizers prevent water loss and make the skin feel softer and smoother. In the study, vitamin E at 5 percent reduced TEWL by 19 percent thirty minutes after application and by

24 percent after four days of twice-daily application. The researcher concluded that vitamin E's efficacy is increased with repeated use.[15]

The claims for vitamin E emollients must be judged in the light of claims for other emollients. Emollients are used for the prevention or relief of dryness, as well as for the protection of the skin. Technically, dryness is a measure of the water content of the skin, and under normal conditions, the water content and vapor pressure of the epidermis are higher than those of the surrounding air. Because of this, water evaporates from the skin surface, excessively so when the skin is exposed to low humidity. Continuous use of soap or detergents or exposure to wind and sun may also increase water loss.

Emollients or "moisturizers" do help make the skin feel softer and smoother. They reduce the roughness, cracking, and irritation of the skin, and they may possibly help to retard the fine wrinkles of aging due to dryness. However, any application of oil to the skin with or without vitamin E replaces a roughened, scaly surface with a smooth film that "cements" down the dry flakes. The oil retards the evaporation of water, but as for the oil penetrating the skin, dermatologists maintain that this is overemphasized. The dryness of the skin is in the layer known as the *stratum corneum,* and it is due to insufficient water in the skin. Emollients keep moisture from evaporating from the skin; they do little to put moisture in.

Most dermatologists say it is the water in emollients, not the oil, that benefits dry skin. Experiments in which a piece of callused skin was placed in oils for as long as three years did not make it flexible again. However, when a brittle piece of callus was placed in water, it soon became flexible.

In the vitamin E experiments performed by Dr. Pugliese, compounds with 1 and 2 percent of vitamin E were not beneficial. It may be that, unlike petrolatum's occlusive effect, which prevents water from evaporating, actual penetration through the skin of vitamin E produces moisturizing from within.[16]

In the 1970s, a major producer of health and beauty aids launched a new underarm deodorant whose "active ingredient" was 4 percent dl-alpha-tocopherol, the alcohol form (natural). This product was thoroughly tested for its potential to cause contact dermatitis and was judged acceptable.

When the product was introduced, many users complained of skin problems, and the product had to be withdrawn from the market.[17] As a result of this experience, considerable concern was generated about the safety of vitamin E.

Vitamin E has a long history of use in cosmetics as an antioxidant to prevent the fatty materials in creams and lotions from going rancid. It is also used to prevent the formation in cosmetics of nitrosamines, powerful cancer-causing agents, which may sometimes occur due to contamination by nitrites.

Bernard Idson, Ph.D., a consultant to the cosmetic industry, writing in *Drug and Cosmetic Industry,* a trade journal, in August 1990, pointed out, "Vitamin E deficiency, irradiation, and aging all lead to much the same kind of damage to cell proteins, membranes, and other structures. The vitamin has been shown to play a role in maintenance of cell membrane integrity, including connective tissue.

"The skin's firmness, texture, or tone are determined by integrity of the elastic fiber in the dermis and connective tissue collagen. Wrinkles occur through loss of subcutaneous fat, degeneration of connective tissue collagen, fibers, and fragmenting of elastic fibers. Thus there is derangement of cell membranes with loss of fat. And while it is unlikely that topical application of low levels of vitamin E can affect the deep subepidermal tissue, it is possible that combined systemic and topical vitamin E use may produce visual elastic epidermal changes."[18]

Summing it up, topical vitamin E has been reported to diminish oxidized fats and tissue damage. However, many claims made for vitamin E creams and skin lotions are hard to prove, as are all claims for cosmetics.

German researchers suggested in the *Journal of Molecular Medicine* in 1995, "Many studies document that vitamin E occupies a central position as a highly efficient antioxidant, thereby providing possibilities to decrease the frequency and severity of pathological events in the skin. For this purpose, increased efforts in developing appropriate systemic and local pharmacological preparations of vitamin E are required."[19]

The medications and cosmetics most readily available on the market are creams and lotions containing the alcohol or acetate forms of vitamin E. Some users break open vitamin E capsules meant for ingestion and apply the contents directly to their skin.

Vitamin E capsules most often contain tocopherol, not tocopheryl acetate. As indicated, tocopherol is the least oxidatively stable form of vitamin E, and this instability may result in the formation of chemical-degradation by-products that may contribute to an increased risk of allergic contact dermatitis. The diluent is often unknown and may be a potential sensitizer or irritant. Creams are on the market with vitamin E levels as high as 25 percent, and researchers are beginning to investigate dose responses.

Cosmetics that contain vitamin E may have just enough so they aren't accused of fraud and not enough to be active. The vitamin, however, may certainly benefit the skin if in a sufficient amount in a proper vehicle.

9

VITAMIN E, SEX, AND FERTILITY

Perhaps the greatest "romance" about the biological benefits of vitamin E concerns sexual potency and fertility. According to current books and folklore, vitamin E can make a man a sexual athlete and a woman appealingly responsive and unfailingly fertile.

The human reproductive system depends upon perfect synchronization not only of chemicals, such as vitamins and hormones, and of organs, such as the penis and vagina, but of the emotions as well.

In the female, eggs are produced by sex glands, the ovaries, which also produce hormones. A hormone is a chemical substance formed in one organ or part of the body and carried in the blood to another organ or part of the body that the hormone arouses to activity.

When ovulation occurs, the egg cell leaves the ovary and is drawn into the opening of one of the two fallopian tubes. One end of each fallopian tube opens near an ovary; this provides a passageway through which the egg cell is carried to the uterus by the motions of fine, hairlike cilia that line the tubes.

The testes are the sex glands of the male and, like the ovaries of women, secrete hormones. Testes also manufacture sperm to fertilize the female's eggs. The testes, which are suspended between the legs in a pouch of skin called the scrotum, are filled with hundreds of fine, threadlike, tightly coiled tubes in which the sperm cells grow.

The penis hangs in front of the testes. The urethra runs the length of the penis and provides a channel through which sperm cells leave the body. For the sperm cells to reach the urethra, they must undergo a complex and hazardous journey. All of the small coiled tubules in one testis open into one larger tube, through which the sperm cells leave their place of manufacture. In the scrotum, behind each testis, this larger tube forms a mass of coils that may serve as a temporary storage space for the sperm cells.

To have intercourse, the man's penis must fill with blood and become erect; the female's vagina must become lubricated and prepared for the penis. For conception to occur from sexual intercourse, perfect synchronization of the release of hormones, egg, and sperm must occur, and the uterus must be in a condition to allow the implantation of the fertilized egg.

With all the new research on oxidized fat causing the buildup of plaque in the heart, brain, and blood vessels, it stands to reason that plaque buildup may interfere with the blood flow to the penis needed for erection. Vitamin E helps the blood carry oxygen to body tissues. It reportedly helps prevent spasms of blood vessels. How much use vitamin E can be in impotence has been a subject of study and controversy.

While there has been little scientific literature on the effect of vitamin E and impotence, the Germans do have one interesting study reported. Urologists at the University of Krefeld Clinic gave impotent men a drug, Afrodor 2000, which is a special mixture of sedatives, aphrodisiacs, and vitamin E. The physicians concluded that the drug is useful for patients with erectile dysfunction of psychological origin.[1]

Definitive, carefully controlled studies have not been done.

There is that unmeasurable factor—the effect of mind on matter. If a man thinks it works, it may. So what is the difference? The result is the same.

HELP WITH INFERTILITY

There has been a lot more research on vitamin E's effect on infertility than on impotence.

The first known effect of vitamin E was the correction of infertility in the female rat. The two scientists who discovered vitamin E, Dr. Herbert M. Evans and Dr. Katherine S. Bishop, found that female rats given diets of rancid lard conceived in a normal manner but reabsorbed the fetus. When they were given a diet containing vitamin E, the problem was corrected.

However, male rats made sterile by lack of vitamin E in the diet could not have their sterility corrected by the addition of tocopherols to their diet.

Since Drs. Evans and Bishop's experiments in the early 1920s, vitamin E deficiency has been found to cause reproductive failure in the female rat, hen, and turkey, and sterility in the male rat, guinea pig, hamster, dog, and rooster. But can findings concerning animals be applied to human beings?

The answer may lie in children with cystic fibrosis, a hereditary disease affecting the pancreas, respiratory system, and sweat glands. These children usually died in childhood, but now, with antibiotics, nebulizers, and other intensive treatments, they may live to adulthood and even marry.

Females with this disease are capable of bearing children, but the males are sterile.

Dr. Carolyn Denning and her associates at Columbia University carried out semen analyses of eight adult male patients with mild, well-controlled cases of cystic fibrosis. The average volume of semen they ejaculated was small, and spermatozoa could not be found in any sample. Blood levels of vitamin E were very low in seven of eight patients. When two of these cases were treated with 300 mg of vitamin E daily, the level of vitamin E in their blood rose to normal values, but analyses of their semen did not show any change.

The Columbia researchers could not explain the absence of sperm. When they examined the tissue from the testicles of ten adult male cystic fibrosis victims, they found evidence of active manufacture of sperm in all, although there were abnormal changes in both the sperm and the tubes that carried the sperm. The defect causing the sterility, the researchers believe, may lie in the transport of sperm out of the testes, the chemical composition of the semen, or a failure to produce enough mature sperm with normal motility. Other researchers have found nothing unusual in the testicular tissue of cystic fibrotic children age five to fifteen, suggesting that the changes may become manifest only after puberty.

A great deal of research is now in progress to determine vitamin E's effect on human sperm. Researchers have found oxygen damage to unsaturated fatty acids in the sperm membrane, which plays a key role in male infertility. In fact, this has been cited as a major cause of men's sterility.[2] Many researchers are now attempting to see if the antioxidants, such as vitamin E, vitamin C, and selenium, can be used to counteract this oxygen damage.

The final results are not in, but some researchers are enthusiastic. In the United Kingdom, investigators at Jessop Hospital for Women, Sheffield, gave 600 mg of vitamin E each day or a placebo to infertile men for three months. The vitamin E pills "significantly improved" the function of the men's sperm.[3]

Canadian researchers are studying whether a combination of the trace mineral selenium and vitamin E could work together to help infertile men. They gave men who were not producing active sperm six months of treatment with selenium and vitamin E. They compared the results to a four-month period before the men took the supplements. Investigators from the University of Montreal's Department of Obstetrics and Gynecology reported significantly improved sperm motility. When the supplements were stopped, the men's sperm returned to the inactivity exhibited before selenium and vitamin E intake. However, during the period of supplementation, none of the couples reported a pregnancy. The researchers are continuing to investigate how vitamin E and selenium improve sperm motility.[4]

Physicians in the Department of Urology at the Cleveland Clinic Foundation, Ohio, cautioned that "the overt commercial claims of antioxidant benefits and supplements for fertility purposes must be cautiously looked into, until proper multicenter clinical trials are studied. From the current data it appears that no single adjuvant will be able to enhance the fertilizing capacity of sperm in infertile men, and a combination of the possible strategies that are not toxic at the dosage used would be a feasible approach."[5]

What about women?

The possibility that vitamin E may affect hormones necessary for reproduction was suggested by Dr. Myron Brin of

Hoffmann–La Roche. Dr. Brin, who was the associate director of vitamin research, pointed out that vitamin E has been found to normalize hormones and improve the clinical condition of women who have cystic mastitis (benign, fluid-filled growths in their breasts). Cystic mastitis can be made better or worse by taking the birth control pill, which contains the female hormones estrogen and progesterone; this reinforces the observations of vitamin E's mediating role in the manufacture of sex hormones.

Fibrocystic breast disease is a benign, though often painful, condition resulting from excessive growth of connective tissue. In a study of twenty-six patients and five controls who received 300 mg of vitamin E per day for two months (following one month of placebo supplementation), interesting results were obtained. Objective and subjective remission was achieved in 85 percent of the patients after treatment. The same laboratory did not find evidence of a beneficial effect of the vitamin in a larger, more controlled study. Another group of investigators found a similar lack of efficacy in treatment of fibrocystic breast disease with vitamin E.[6]

In earlier work, however, Dr. S. C. Sommers of Boston University found that women with cystic mastitis have an abnormality of the lining of the uterus, the thyroid gland, the ovaries, and the pituitary gland. All of these conditions involve the metabolism of hormones. Cystic mastitis suggests a hormonal imbalance. When Dr. Sommers measured hormone levels in urine, he found them abnormal in women with cystic mastitis. When he gave vitamin E, he found four out of six women then had normal hormone levels in the urine, and their cystic mastitis was cured.

While it has not been proven in well-controlled studies that vitamin E helps protect women from mastitis—inflammation of the breast—in cows, both vitamin E and selenium, its trace metal partner, have long been used to protect their udders from it.[7]

There does seem to be an almost certain benefit from vitamin E for women on the pill. Supplements of 200 IU a day reduced platelet activity in women on oral contraceptives. Platelets are blood cells that are key elements in clotting. Supplements of 400 IU a day inhibited in platelet adhesion to collagen in healthy adults. These effects on platelet function suggest a role for vitamin E in the prevention of blood clots.[8]

While there may be exaggerated claims for vitamin E and sexual function, remember, the name itself—*tocopherol*—means to bring forth childbirth.

10

VITAMIN E AGAINST AGING

As we age, the concentration of vitamin E in our tissues decreases, as do a lot of other substances.[1] As a result, we lose some protection against the damage to our cells by those old devils, free radicals.

Denham Harman, D.C., Ph.D., professor of biochemistry at the University of Nebraska and founder of AGE, the American Aging Association, believes that vitamin E deficiency, radiation damage, and aging have a common link—impairment or destruction of the cell caused by free radicals.

In studies at the University of Nebraska, Dr. Harman demonstrated that exposure of lab animals to radiation appeared to rapidly age the animals and caused an increase in free-radical levels in their cells.[2] Research has also documented the progressive accumulation of lipofuscin (age pigments) in aging in every animal species studied.[3]

Increased cancer with advancing age may be due at least in part to the increasing level of free-radical reactions with age, along with the diminishing ability of the immune system to eliminate damaged cells. In cancer, the mechanism of the cell goes haywire and the cell grows out of control; in aging, the mechanism of the cell works less efficiently or not at all. A substance that could keep the cell's components in proper working order could control or prevent both cancer and aging. A number of eminent scientists think that substance is vitamin E.

As pointed out in prior chapters, researchers are reporting that people who consume a lot of vitamin E have less cardio-vascular disease and cancer than others. To find out whether the vitamin has more general antiaging effects, Drs. Jeff E. Poulin and Marguerite M. B. Kay and their colleagues at the University of Arizona College of Medicine fed aging mice three different diets:

- normal
- high in vitamin E
- high in beta-carotene (which is converted in the body into vitamin A)

Then they examined *band 3 proteins* in the rodents' brain and immune-system cells.[4] These vital proteins are found in all mammalian cells, including ours. They hold cells together and regulate key biological processes. They are among the first proteins to break down in aging. Because band 3 proteins weave like an undulating snake through the membranes of cells, they are vulnerable to both free radicals formed *inside* cells during normal metabolism and to free radicals *outside* cells that are acquired from elsewhere in the body and carried in body fluids. Their destruction appears to be a defining step of cell aging and death.

The Arizona researchers concluded that vitamin E sup-plements, in amounts equivalent to a human dose of about 400 IUs a day, could prolong the life of cells by preventing or delaying oxidative damage to band 3 proteins.

After seven months, the Arizona team found middle-aged mice on the high vitamin E diet retained twice the band 3 function in their immune system cells as did their counterparts on a normal diet. Older mice on the vitamin E diet experienced none of the destructive band 3 changes in brain cells that normally lead to those cells' demise. There were no effects in the beta-carotene group.

Dr. Kay says she studied cells in the brain and immune systems because these two systems influence all other cells and organs in the body. She added that these systems are also the most affected by aging. Cells in both the brain and the immune system, which perform the most complex functions such as thinking and encoding memory and recognizing and attacking foreign invaders, are the first to go.

"A lot of vitamin knowledge tends to be anecdotal, almost old wives' tales," said Dr. Kay. "But now we have actually a sensible molecular base to show that vitamin E is in fact doing a number of good things. Now we have clinical proof."

The amounts of vitamin E found protective in laboratory studies—from 100 to 400 IU—cannot be achieved through a normal diet, particularly a diet that is low in fat. The results strengthen the case that vitamin E can slow age-related cellular decay, Dr. Kay said. But she warned that more than 1,000 IU of vitamin E per day can be toxic.

IMMUNITY, AGING, AND VITAMIN E

Our immune system is complex. It wasn't so long ago that scientists first realized that we have an immune system just as we have nervous, gastrointestinal, and cardiovascular systems. In the 1960s, they found the immune system is a widely distributed whole-body network that includes the lymph nodes, spleen, tonsils, thymus gland, bone marrow, and white blood cells. These organs are in total communication with each other, and they are, in ways as yet not fully understood, orchestrated.

When the system is operating at its optimal level, our defenses are in harmony and we are protected against all sorts of potential enemies from the common cold to cancer. If our immune instruments don't play in concert, we become ill. If one or more elements overreact or play an off note, we develop allergies or arthritis or some other malady in which our cells attack our own bodies.

The "music" for our immune system is very much influenced by what we eat.

It has been known for many years that if we have a large deficiency of certain vitamins and nutrients, we will become ill and die. The association between malnutrition and lowered disease resistance is taken for granted. It is also well accepted that children and older adults do not have as strong an immune system as young adults. But what about subclinical deficiencies that may affect our health in subtle ways? Is it possible that genetic facts make some of us less able to use certain elements in our food necessary to our well-being?

With the discovery of penicillin and other antimicrobial agents, beginning in the 1940s, medicine entered the antibiotic era. Because of the effectiveness of these new therapeutic agents, plus a plethora of other exciting breakthroughs, interest in the nutritional aspects of host resistance and immunology began to fade.[5] Then in 1975, the subcommittee on Nutrition and Infection of the National Academy of Science National Research Council extended its review process to cover the topic of malnutrition and the immune system. Several years later, the Nutritional Advisory Board of the American Medical Association sponsored a small workshop to review the immunological effects provided by single essential trace nutrients.

In the 1980s and 1990s, prodded by the expense of traditional medicines and the desire of the public to have more "natural remedies," and a greater understanding of human physiology, the research on vitamins and other nutrients began to pick up steam. Roadblocks occurred because few scientists were trained in both vitamin research and immunology. It was also difficult to produce vitamin-deficiency states in many species of laboratory animals.[6]

Can vitamin E and other antioxidants help to rejuvenate the aging immune system?

The immune response of elderly individuals tends to decline, as demonstrated by decreased proliferation of white blood cells, delayed type hypersensitivity skin testing, and decreased interleukin-2 production. Interleukin, a natural substance occurring in the body, transmits signals between types of white blood cells. Interleukin-2 has been used to fight cancers, and to stimulate immunity in patients with AIDS.

Simin N. Meydani, D.V.M., Ph.D., of the USDA Human Nutrition Research Center on Aging at Tufts University in Boston, recruited thirty-four healthy volunteers over the age of sixty who moved into a metabolic research dormitory at the USDA Human Nutrition Center for thirty days.[7] Half of the volunteers received a normal diet containing about 15 IU of vitamin E. The other half received the same diet but also took two capsules daily containing a total of 800 IU of vitamin E.

The immune response was measured at the beginning and the end of the thirty-day study. Those who received vitamin

E had a "significant increase" in immune function. The cells of the immune system are among the most sensitive in the body to oxidation. Thus, they are the first to be affected as the body's normal repair processes begin to fail with age. Vitamin E is an antioxidant. It tracks down the reactive form of oxygen and defangs it so that it can no longer cause damage. It can also stimulate the action of immune system components that are themselves antioxidants.

Dr. Meydani performed yet another study at the USDA Human Nutrition Research Center on Aging. Her recent work in animals and humans showed that the body's immune response is compromised when a diet is deficient in vitamins E and B_6.[8] She found this depressed immune function was corrected by supplementation with vitamins E and B_6. She says maintenance of optimal immune response in the elderly may require supplementation of vitamins E and B_6 at levels higher than the RDA.

In still another study reported in the May 7, 1997, issue of the *Journal of the American Medical Association,* Dr. Meydani and her colleagues at the Jean Mayer USDA Human Nutrition Research Center on Aging at Tufts University, reported good results with vitamin E alone. They gave 60, 200, or 800 mg of vitamin E for 235 days to 88 healthy elderly people living in the community. The results indicated that a level of vitamin E greater than currently recommended enhances immunity in healthy elderly persons. No adverse effects were observed.

Dr. Meydani and others believe that the body does not get enough vitamin E in a normal diet to efficiently combat oxidation. About 60 percent of the vitamin E in our foods comes from vegetable oils, such as margarines, salad dressings, and shortenings. As we try to reduce fat in our diet to lower the risk of heart disease and cancer, these are the first items to go.

ALZHEIMER'S AND DOWN'S AND VITAMIN E

Is the central control of aging of the whole body located in the brain? Support for this theory can be found in Down's syndrome, a genetic abnormality that involves mental retardation and certain physical characteristics such as eyes that slant upward, short hands, and a stubby nose. Down's syndrome individuals die earlier than psychotics or normal adults. They have eighteen times the incidence of leukemia and twenty-six times the incidence of cancer as the population at large. They also go bald in childhood and develop wrinkled skin at an early age. They are born with broken chromosomes. The rest of us acquire broken chromosomes as we go along.

The cells of Down's syndrome individuals produce more free radicals, and their cells contain more rancid fats (lipid peroxidation), which poses a potential risk for tissue damage.

In a study at the Brain-Behavior Research Center of the University of California at San Francisco, researchers sought to determine the level of vitamin E and vitamin A in circulation and correlate it with oxidized fat in the Down's condition. The results obtained from twelve Down's and twelve normal subjects indicated that Down's syndrome is associated with significant decreases in plasma and red blood cell levels of vitamins A and E and significant increases in oxidized fat in red blood cells. This is a result of the increased rancid fat depleting the antioxidant vitamins. When A and E are depleted, oxygen damage to tissue occurs.[9]

In a related study conducted in Britain, plasma vitamin E levels measured in twelve Down's syndrome subjects with

Alzheimer's disease were lower than in twelve Down's syndrome subjects without it. Alzheimer's is a deterioration of the brain with severe memory impairment. Down's syndrome individuals are at high risk for developing it as early as twenty or thirty years of age. One explanation for this, again, is that the excess of free radicals causes oxidative damage and accounts for the premature aging.

In Alzheimer's disease, there are characteristic nerve tangles and amyloid deposits. Amyloid is a protein substance in tissues and organs that are degenerating. When excessive amyloid builds up on the brain, it interferes with the brain's nerve network, disrupting normal function. Some researchers believe it is oxidation that causes the buildup of amyloid that eventually leads to Alzheimer's.[10]

In disease states where the body's use of fat is impaired, a clinical picture of cell malfunctioning involving such deposits is clear. The relationship between vitamin E and cystic fibrosis—a hereditary disease usually affecting the pancreas, respiratory system, and sweat glands—has been intensively studied since 1956 when Dr. Ella H. Oppenheimer, a Johns Hopkins pathologist, found an infant with localized muscle lesions similar to the kind found in vitamin E deficient animals. This led researchers at Columbia University in New York to review the autopsy findings of 151 cases of cystic fibrosis victims. Ceroid deposits—brown, waxlike pigments—often heavy, were found in the intestinal tract and other tissues of every child over the age of two. Later, an accumulation of ceroid deposits was found in the central nervous systems of six patients who had died of the disease.

In children with cystic fibrosis, researchers wanted to determine which level of vitamin E supplementation was appropriate. They took blood samples from the children before and after one year of supplementation with either 15 IU or 100 IU per day of vitamin E. Before, all the children had low blood levels of vitamin E. When twelve months had passed, the researchers discovered the vitamin E in the red blood cells had risen to normal levels in those youngsters on the 100-IU-per-day vitamin E supplement but not in those on the 15-IU supplement.[11]

The same type of ceroid deposits seen in cystic fibrosis and other vitamin E deficient conditions were found in the elderly as far back as 1894. It was noted then that nerve cells of the unborn child contained no pigment, but the cells of the senile elderly were clogged with it.

An authority on vitamin E, Dr. David Herting, formerly of Eastman Kodak, a large distiller of the nutrient, said at a science writers seminar sponsored by the Vitamin Information Bureau on June 5, 1968, that the accumulation of ceroid pigment in smooth muscles in patients unable to absorb fat is similar to that in aged men and rats and is apparently irreversible.

However, vitamin E deficiency produces an even greater accumulation of ceroid in the nerve cells of young rats than is found in senile nondeficient rats and may therefore be an important factor contributing to the deposition of ceroid pigments in the nerve cells of man.

Since some studies show that vitamin E protects against oxidative damage, the hope is that it might protect against or slow down the development of Alzheimer's-like dementia in those with Down's.[12] In one study, however, vitamin E in the brains of Alzheimer's patients was not lower than in those of patients without Alzheimer's.[13]

Multicenter research is now under way to study the effects of vitamin E supplementation in Alzheimer's disease. Again, the emphasis is on determining if vitamin E can prevent oxidative damage in brain cells.[14] Exciting results have already been reported. In the April 24, 1997, issue of the *New England Journal of Medicine* researchers funded by The National Institutes of Health determined that daily administration of 2,000 IU of vitamin E, 10 milligrams of selegiline (a drug that boosts the neurotransmitter, dopamine), or a combination of the two slowed functional deterioration in moderately severe Alzheimer's patients. The two-year study included 341 patients recruited from 35 academic medical centers actively involved in Alzheimer's research.

"For the first time we are seeing research findings that offer hope for potential agents that may halt the progression of AD, rather than agents that provide symptomatic relief of the cognitive loss in AD," reported Mary Sano, Ph.D., College of Physicians & Surgeons, Columbia University, New York, who directed the research effort.

Dr. Ishwarlal Jialal, M.D., associate professor of pathology and internal medicine at the University of Texas Southwestern Medical Center at Dallas and a leading vitamin E researcher, commented on the study: "Anyone with a family history of Alzheimer's disease or heart disease would be foolish not to take daily vitamin E supplements."

Dr. Kay, the University of Arizona researcher whose band 3 protein study was described earlier, believes that vitamin E could also help protect against Alzheimer's in healthy adults since it protects the vital band 3 proteins in both the immune and nervous systems.[15]

PARKINSON'S DISEASE

Does the environment cause neurological disorders such as Alzheimer's disease and Parkinson's disease? Can a toxic environment play an important role in initiating the disease years before symptoms appear?[16] Parkinson's, a chronic neurologic disease of unknown cause, is characterized by tremors, rigidity, and abnormal gait. Does oxygen damage to cells caused by environmental factors contribute to the development of parkinsonism? If so, then antioxidants such as vitamin E may be effective in early treatment of the disease.[17]

Although animal studies of chemically induced parkinsonism showed no improvement or prevention with high-dose vitamin E administration, a preliminary human trial was encouraging, and some patients with Parkinson's disease who were self-supplementing with vitamin E reportedly had significantly less severe disease symptoms than matched controls.[18]

In addition, patients with tardive dyskinesia showed some improvement on vitamin E. This disorder is caused by long-term use of certain tranquilizers and other drugs that affect the brain. One of the theories is that the uncontrolled movements associated with the disorder may be the result of oxidation damage to nerve endings. A controlled study of fifteen patients with tardive dyskinesia was conducted with 1,200 IU of a tocopherol for two-week periods. The supplemented group exhibited a 43 reduction in scores on an abnormal involuntary-movement test. The scores of patients not on vitamin E were not significantly changed.[19]

Therefore, in 1987, there was heightened enthusiasm when a multicenter controlled clinical trial of deprenyl, which inhibits a brain chemical involved in depression (monoamine oxidase), and vitamin E in the treatment of early Parkinson's disease got under way.[20] Eight hundred patients were randomly assigned to one of four treatments: placebo, active tocopherol and deprenyl placebo, active deprenyl and tocopherol placebo, or both active drugs. An interim analysis showed that deprenyl was beneficial.

The beneficial effects of deprenyl, which occurred largely during the first twelve months of treatment, remained strong and significantly delayed the onset of disability for an average of about nine months. The high dose of vitamin E (2,000 IU per day) was not effective.[21]

Still, nerve and muscle abnormalities are associated with vitamin E deficiencies. The mechanism of action of vitamin E is assumed to be through antioxidant protection of membranes and/or membranes' stabilization. It has been suggested that the large surface area of certain nerves is particularly susceptible to oxidative damage.[22] And perhaps new studies at a different dosage or in combination with something else will demonstrate that vitamin E can be beneficial in the treatment of Parkinson's.

CATARACTS

A cataract is an opacity of the lens of the eye. Babies may be born with cataracts, but most cataracts are associated with aging. The opacity gradually occurs with increasing age, physical or chemical injury, diabetes, and other endocrine diseases. The only way to restore useful vision is to remove the lens surgically; this permits light waves to enter the eye once again.

Can vitamin E help prevent cataracts?

Cataracts are caused, in part, by the oxidation of lens proteins. Exposure to ultraviolet light is thought to be one of the causes of oxidation, and cataracts are more common in countries that have strong sunlight through most of the year. The lens of the eye contains a high concentration of vitamin C, glutathione, and antioxidant enzymes, presumably to provide protection against ultraviolet-light-induced oxidative damage. As pointed out, levels of all antioxidants in the body decline with age, and the risk of developing cataracts increases with age.[23] A number of studies have shown people suffering from cataracts have lower levels of the antioxidant nutrients in their systems.[24]

In an epidemiological study on cataract risk in adults older than fifty-five, for example, investigators at the University of Western Ontario in Toronto found a statistically significant protective effect of vitamin E along with vitamin C. In the Canadian study, cataract risk was compared in people taking vitamin E and vitamin C supplements and in people taking no supplements. For the vitamin E, the unsupplemented group had a two and a half times greater risk than the supplement takers; for vitamin C, the unsupplemented group had a fourfold greater risk than the supplement takers.[25]

Unlike previous studies, which relied on diet surveys, a Finnish study published in the December 1992 issue of the *British Medical Journal* measured levels of nutrients in the blood.[26]

Dr. Paul Knekt, the leading investigator at the Social Insurance Institute in Helsinki, said the findings showed a "strong link" between low nutrient levels and the likelihood of needing cataract surgery. But he said further studies were needed to prove that diet could decrease the risk of getting cataracts.

Harvard Medical School researchers then reported in the May 1994 issue of the *American Journal of Public Health* that they had conducted a study to examine prospectively the association between reported use of vitamin supplements and the risk of cataract and cataract extraction.[27]

The participants were 17,744 American male doctors forty to eighty-four years old in the Physicians' Health Study. Those who in 1982 did not report they had cataracts and provided complete information about vitamin supplementation and other risk factors were followed for sixty months. During that time, there were 370 cataracts and 109 cataract extractions.

When the study compared physicians who took multivitamins to those who did not use any supplements, those who took the vitamins had a relative risk of cataract of 0.73 after adjustment for other risk factors. For cataract extraction, the corresponding relative risk was 0.79. Use of the antioxidant vitamins C and/or vitamin E supplements alone was not associated with a reduced risk of cataract, but the size of this subgroup was small. The researchers concluded that the men who took multivitamin supplements tended to experience a decreased risk of cataract, and they said there is a need for rigorous testing of this hypothesis in large-scale randomized trials in men and women.

People with a low level of vitamin A and vitamin E, according to a Finnish study, are nearly twice as likely to need cataract surgery as those with high levels. Several other studies have had similar results that appear to support the hypothesis that protecting the lens from oxygen damage with antioxidant vitamins may help defend against cataract development.[28]

Should you get your antioxidant vitamins in food rather than in supplements to prevent cataracts?

In a 1995 study, Julie A. Mares-Perlman, Ph.D., assistant professor of ophthalmology and visual sciences at the Center for Health Sciences University of Wisconsin-Madison found that certain whole foods may be more important than individual nutrients in prevention of nuclear sclerosis, an early stage of one form of cataract. She says, "My message to the scientific community and to the general public is to focus on eating nutritious foods in and of themselves rather than specific nutrients because we don't know for certain what is providing the benefit.[29]

Dr. Mares-Perlman measured the amount of three common antioxidants in foods and multivitamin supplements: carotenoids and vitamins C and E. She then examined the overall intake of these antioxidants in people with and without early cataracts. Although researchers expected those with diets rich in antioxidants would have a lower rate of early cataracts, this wasn't the case. Rather, results showed men and women consuming the highest total of these specific nutrients didn't have a lower rate of early cataracts than those with a smaller intake.

When whole foods were considered, however, the picture was different. Men consuming the highest amounts of vegetables, particularly green ones, were less likely to have early cataracts. This pattern persisted even after adjusting for age and history of smoking and drinking, all of which are associated with cataracts. Mares-Perlman said this preliminary finding indicates that overall intake of certain foods may be more crucial in avoiding some types of cataracts and possibly other diseases than specific antioxidant nutrients.

Among women, higher intake of vegetables wasn't related to the frequency of early cataracts even though women generally ate more vegetables than men did. While the reason for the disparity is unknown, Dr. Mares-Perlman said men may benefit more from certain food components because of their higher incidence of smoking, alcohol consumption, and exposure to occupational pollutants. Alternatively, it may be more difficult to detect protective relationships with foods in women. When studying cataracts, which tend to develop over many years, diet histories may be less accurate in women, who tend to change eating behavior more than men over time.

A strong association was found with fruit and vegetable intake: people who ate 3.5 or more servings of fruits and vegetables daily had a much lower risk of developing cataracts than people who ate 1.5 servings or less.[30]

Allen Taylor, Ph.D., director of the Laboratory for Nutrition and Vision Research at the USDA Human Nutrition Research Center on Aging in Boston, says antioxidant nutrients (vitamins C and E, and beta-carotene, a plant-based precursor for vitamin A) appear to protect the eye from damage caused by light and oxygen. They may also help maintain the eye's ability to get rid of damaged proteins that can exacerbate the development of cataracts. "The protection offered by antioxidant nutrients could play a part in reducing the incidence of lens cataracts and other leading causes of blindness in aging," Taylor says.

In a review of the evidence on cataracts and nutrition, Dr. Taylor commented that the antioxidant nutrients may provide a means to "delay the onset of cataract in the underdeveloped countries" and in developed countries to "impede further the rate at which cataract develops." Because of the sharply increased prevalence of cataracts after age seventy-five, "it is estimated that the need for cataract extractions would be diminished by half if onset of cataract could be delayed by only ten years."[31]

Such a ten-year delay might eliminate the need for half of the 1.4 million yearly lens extractions in the United States. At over $3 billion, expenses for cataract-related problems and lens extractions are the largest line item in the Medicare budget.

MACULAR DEGENERATION

Another eye problem that afflicts older persons is macular degeneration, the leading cause of irreversible blindness in the United States.[32] The macula, the area of the retina near the optic nerve at the back of the eye, is the part of the eye that distinguishes fine detail at the center of the field of vision. In some elderly people, the small blood vessels of the eye become constricted or narrowed and hardened. As a result, the macula is starved for blood and degenerates. An estimated 25 percent of people over sixty-five have some manifestation of this disease.[33]

Since vitamin E helps blood vessels stay healthy and aids in defending against oxygen damage, will it help stave off macular degeneration?

Johanna Seddon, M.D., from the Epidemiology Unit, Massachusetts Eye and Ear Infirmary, and Charles H. Hennekens, M.D., a prime researcher on diet and disease, consider published studies regarding vitamins, minerals, and macular degeneration "important and promising," but at present insufficient to support a clinical recommendation.[34] The doctors note, "There are several caveats to consider before treating eye disease with vitamin and mineral supplements at this time. In the United States, most people prefer prescription of preventive agent more than proscription of harmful lifestyles. It would be unfortunate if the elderly took supplements while continuing to smoke or while not complying with therapy for hypertension, both of which appear to be associated with advanced macular degeneration.

"In addition, what dose should be taken or how long should they be taken to demonstrate any effect? It is plausible that the intake of antioxidant-rich foods is protective, but the benefit may result not from their antioxidant properties but from some other component that these foods have in common. Antioxidant supplements in that particular circumstance would not be helpful.

"It is imperative," Drs. Seddon and Hennekens state, "that we do find answers to the questions concerning the effects of antioxidants, if any, since these agents represent potentially beneficial treatment for a common and serious eye disease. Fortunately, reliable data on which to base public health recommendations are already accumulating from large-scale randomized trials. At present, the hypothesis regarding antioxidant therapy for AMD (age-related macular degeneration) is promising, but far from proven."

One of the respected studies providing clues to the use of antioxidants against AMD is the Baltimore Longitudinal Study of Aging, supported by the U.S. National Institute on Aging. The relationships between fasting blood levels of vitamins A, C, and E and beta-carotene and AMD were studied. The data were collected two or more years before assessment of macular status.[35]

A total of 976 participants were in the study at Johns Hopkins Medical Institutions, Baltimore, Maryland. The data suggest a protective effect against AMD for high plasma values of vitamin E. An antioxidant index composed of plasma vitamin C, vitamin E, and beta-carotene was also protective.

The eye researchers said their conclusions must be tempered with the knowledge that the population under study was basically well nourished, and few individuals had any clinically deficient states. They noted, "The study cannot exclude the possibility that quite low levels of micronutrients, lower than those observed, in this study, might be risk factors for AMD."

Yet, the researchers concluded that the use of vitamin supplements to prevent AMD was not supported by the data.

The final answer is not in yet. The Eye Disease Case-Control Study Group supported by the National Eye Institute had this conclusion about antioxidants and AMD:

"We evaluated the hypothesis that higher serum levels of micronutrients with antioxidant capabilities may be associated with a decreased risk of neovascular age-related macular degeneration by comparing serum levels of carotenoids, vitamin C and vitamin E, and selenium in 421 patients with neovascular age-related macular degeneration and 615 controls. Subjects were classified by blood levels of the micronutrient (low, medium, and high). Persons with carotenoid levels in the medium and high groups, compared with those in the low group, had markedly reduced risks of neovascular age-related macular degeneration, with levels of risk reduced to one-half and one-third, respectively. Although no statistically significant protective effect was found for vitamin C or vitamin E or selenium individually, an antioxidant index that combined all four micronutrient measurements showed statistically significant reductions of risk with increasing levels of the index. Although these results suggest that higher blood levels of micronutrients with antioxidant potential, in particular, carotenoids, may be associated with a decreased risk of the most visually disabling form of age-related macular degeneration, it would be premature to translate these findings into nutritional recommendations."[36]

ARTHRITIS

Animal research has demonstrated the effectiveness of vitamin E supplementation in inhibiting the elevation of free-radical concentrations associated with arthritis.[37] A double-blind study of patients with osteoarthritis also showed that vitamin E was significantly superior to a placebo for pain relief, necessity of additional analgesic medication, and improved mobility.[38]

In one study, 400 IU of alpha tocopherol was given daily for six weeks to patients suffering from arthritis. The patients were reportedly able to reduce their use of painkillers, particularly nonsteroidal anti-inflammatory drugs (NSAID). Such drugs may have serious side effects such as bleeding. One vitamin E pill of 400 IU is considered harmless.[39]

Multicenter research to determine vitamin E's antioxidant, anti-inflammatory potential in arthritic joints is under way at this writing. Dr. Vishwa Singh, head of human-nutrition research at Hoffman–La Roche, one of the major producers of vitamin E, notes, "Inflammation and free radicals are linked and produce joint damage."[40]

Aside from its potential as an anti-inflammatory substance, vitamin E may actually have an effect on bone. In reportedly one of the first studies to show vitamin E's importance in bone growth, Purdue University researchers found that supplemental vitamin E supports bone growth. Food scientist and nutritionist Bruce Watkins and bone biologist Mark Seifert, associate professor at Purdue's School of Medicine, found that when chicks were given extra vitamin E, the rate of bone formation in the spongy ends of leg bones was greater than in chicks not given the supplement. It also suggests, they say, that vitamin E protects against cellular fat rancidity in cartilage to sustain normal bone growth and model-ing.[41]

"Our research may have implications in reducing risk for osteoporosis, if vitamin E reduces bone breakdown and enhances bone formation," Watkins says. "Also, vitamin E has been used with some success in reducing the severity of inflammatory arthritis in the elderly."

VITAMIN E REDUCES MORTALITY

Can vitamin E with its powers to fight oxygen damage actually prolong life?

Dr. Denham Harman of the University of Nebraska, a pioneer gerontologist and founder of the American Aging Association, believed that by adding vitamin E or some other equally effective antioxidant to the diet, the useful life span of humans could be increased by five to ten years.[42]

"In any given individual," Dr. Harman said, "the increase in the duration of useful life would be expected to be greater the younger the person at the time the free-radical approach is started. This is not to say the application of this method to persons in the later part of their life span might not have significant benefits."

Dr. Harman was able to prolong the lives of rats dying of amyloidosis, a condition that is frequently found in aging humans. It is characterized by the accumulation of abnormal protein fibers in the organs. It is always accompanied by anemia and occurs in a variety of illnesses including chronic infections (such as tuberculosis), liver disease, and of course in "aging."

Canadian scientists in 1996 reported that the life span of the female flies fed vitamin E did indeed increase. They found that antioxidant enzymes were positively linked to the longer-lived insects.[43]

Dr. Aloys Tappel, professor of Food Science and Technology at the University of California, Dr. Harman, and other researchers have been able to prolong the life of animals by giving them vitamin E, but to reproduce the same experiments in humans would be difficult. Dr. Harman and Dr. Tappel among others have believed since the early 1970s that by adding vitamin E or some other equally effective antioxidant to the diet, the useful life span of humans could be increased by five to ten years.

Is there any scientific evidence? Yes, and it comes from a large government-financed study.

An epidemiologic study of 11,178 people over sixty-five was conducted by the National Institute on Aging.[44] Vitamin E supplements were reported to lower total mortality rates by 27 percent, reduce the risk of heart disease mortality by 41 percent, and decrease cancer mortality by 22 percent. The study looked at the association between the use of vitamin E and vitamin C supplements and all causes of mortality. It was based on an analysis of data from the Established Populations for Epidemiologic Studies of the Elderly, a compilation of health and disease data collected from four communities of people from 65 to 105 years old. The respondents were followed for six years with mortality data available for an additional two to three years.

The data analysis did not include the dosage of vitamin supplements taken or the duration over which they were consumed. The researchers did note that the amounts in individual supplements of vitamin E tend to be more than 100 IU and individual supplements of vitamin C are likely to include higher doses than in multiple vitamins.

The researchers noted that vitamin C supplements alone had no effect on the risk of death. Simultaneous use of vitamin E and vitamin C supplements was associated with a 42 percent lower risk of total mortality and a 53 percent lower risk of coronary mortality. Multiple vitamin/mineral supplements and other supplements had no effect on mortality risk. Why did the use of multiple vitamin/mineral supplements and other supplements have no effect on mortality risk? This finding was explained by the fact that "while a multiple vitamin/mineral supplement may contain some vitamin E, the concentrations may not be high enough to be protective."

The researchers speculate the findings are due to the ability of vitamin E to stabilize free radicals that cause conditions linked to heart disease, including oxidation of LDL (see glossary). Similarly, they noted that the "lower risk of cancer mortality may be explained by a reduction of free radical damage to DNA, a possible cause of cancer."

Adjustments for alcohol use, smoking history, aspirin taking, and medical conditions did not substantially alter the findings.

"These findings," the government researchers said, "are consistent with those for younger persons and suggest protective effects of vitamin E supplements in the elderly."

These results are consistent with those of the Health Professionals Follow-Up study conducted by Harvard with forty thousand men, forty to seventy-five years old, which found a 39 percent decrease in heart disease risk in those who took at least 100 IU of vitamin E daily from food and supplements. In the recent Cambridge Heart Antioxidant Study (CHAOS) of two thousand men and women, the risk of nonfatal heart attack dropped 75 percent in those who took 400 to 800 IU of vitamin E supplements daily. The Nurses' Health Study of eighty-seven thousand women, thirty-four to fifty-nine years old, found a 40 percent reduction in heart disease in the group with the highest level of vitamin E intake.

There has been great emphasis, fueled by pharmaceutical companies and the government, to lower cholesterol to stave off heart attacks and strokes. Individuals with low cholesterol, however, experience greater than expected mortality from nonatherosclerotic diseases, including cancer and respiratory and digestive illnesses, according to a study by researchers at the University of Pittsburgh.[45]

Antioxidant activity in the blood as well as concentrations of vitamin E and vitamin C were compared in two groups of twenty-four subjects, one with low LDL (bad) cholesterol and low total cholesterol and the other with average cholesterol. The low and average cholesterol groups were equivalent in gender mix, age, weight, and serum total protein. Results reveal that compared with the high group, the low cholesterol group had decreased total serum antioxidant activity. The two groups did not differ in vitamin C. The difference in total antioxidant activity in the blood concentration was greater among men than women. Low cholesterol was associated with reduced absolute vitamin E levels, although the tocopherol:cholesterol ratio was the same in low and high cholesterol individuals. These data indicate that low cholesterol may be associated with low serum antioxidant reserve, possibly increasing susceptibility to oxidation.

Dr. Harman of the University of Nebraska maintains that the destruction of fat by oxygen in living men is the basic deteriorative reaction in the aging cell.[46]

"In human nutrition," he said, "the greatest impact of these findings may come from the resulting increase in the knowledge of lipid peroxidation [the combining of fat with oxygen] in the aging processes. These processes may be a universal disease, the chemical deteriorative effects of which might be slowed by the increased use of dietary antioxidants."

He said these reactions are almost completely suppressed by biological antioxidants, and he pointed out that vitamin E is the only well-known antioxidant that occurs naturally in the covering and lining of the cell.

11

HOW MUCH VITAMIN E
DO YOU NEED?

How much vitamin E do I need? Am I getting enough vitamin E in my diet? Should I take vitamin E supplements? These are the questions asked by those of us who are confused by the controversy over the most mysterious of all the vitamins.

How much vitamin E does it take to

- prevent a deficiency?
- to ward off the oxidation of fat within the body?
- to deter the development of heart disease, cancer, and other ills?

In 1968, the Food and Nutrition Board of the National Research Council, which provides the advice for government standards, acknowledged vitamin E was essential. The U.S. recommended daily allowance (RDA) in 1973 was then set at 30 IU daily for adults. This was intended to be an amount that would allow for increased consumption of polyunsaturated fatty acids. Polyunsaturates are those fats from vegetable sources, which are liquid at room temperature, as opposed to saturated fats from animals, which are usually solid at room temperature. The recognition that saturated fats contribute to the buildup of plaques in the arteries caused government and health organizations to encourage the public to replace saturated fats with unsaturated ones. Unsaturated fats, however, deplete vitamin E. Low-cholesterol or fat-modified diets rich in polyunsaturated fats raise the body's need for vitamin E.

In 1989, nevertheless, the Food and Nutrition Board of the National Research Council lowered the recommended daily allowance for vitamin E to 15 IU for adult males and 12 IU for adult females. Why did the members of the board reduce the amount needed?

The RDAs are designed to meet the basic requirements of healthy people to stave off deficiencies. The expert panel members of the Food and Nutrition Board do not consider environment, lifestyle, or physical and mental conditions that may affect our individual needs. Their reasoning was that, in general, it was unlikely we would be able to obtain as much as 30 IU of vitamin E through our diets.[1]

The intake of vitamin E in our diets, according to government surveys, was 10.4 to 13.4 IU per day in 1989.[2] In government studies ongoing at this writing, according to Dr. Vishwa N. Singh, director of human-nutrition research at Hoffmann–La Roche, the current intake of vitamin E by the general population is 9.8 IU.[3] This is adequate, almost everyone agrees, to prevent vitamin E deficiency in the majority of the population.

Vitamin E deficiency has been blamed in humans for almost everything—from impotence to heart disease, from muscular dystrophy to cancer. This has caused some skepticism among scientists, who cannot believe that so many symptoms could possibly be related to one vitamin. And yet recent studies have shown that vitamin E is essential to every tissue, every single cell, and every membrane in the body.

Drs. F. Weber and H. Weiser, two Swiss researchers, pointed out at a meeting of the New York Academy of Medicine in the 1970s "that we know as yet too little about the effects of vitamin E deficiency on the human organism. For instance, we do not know all of what type of deficiency symptoms could be expected in man, since the vitamin E deficiency in animals is characterized by an exceptional multitude of deficiency manifestations that are also dependent on various factors of nutrition.

"Further," the two researchers said, "it has to be taken into consideration that characteristic and clinically easily recognizable deficiency symptoms often become manifest with an extreme vitamin deficiency only, whereas latent deficiencies, so-called hypovitaminoses, are very difficult to diagnose because of uncharacteristic symptoms. It is possible that vitamin E deficiency in many will produce effects only after a prolonged period of time, for instance, in atherosclerosis or other so-called attrition conditions."

Dr. Max Horwitt of the University of Illinois pointed out at the same academy meeting that in the rat, for instance, it is possible to have apparent good health according to objective standards (such as rate of growth) and still have vitamin E pathology present: "For example, rats on stripped-corn-oil diets continued to grow at near optimum rates for twenty weeks after the onset of creatinuria [excess of creatine excreted in the urine, believed to be a precursor of muscular dystrophy]. Similarly, in humans, there were no significant signs of anemia when the decreased erythrocyte [red blood cell] survival was noted, because of the ability of the blood-forming system to make up the difference."

Since vitamin E is a fat-soluble vitamin, the presence of both bile and fat are required for proper absorption of vitamin E. Absorption takes place in the small intestine where 20 to 30 percent of the intake passes through the intestinal wall into the lymph.[4]

Once absorbed, vitamin E attaches itself to the beta-lipoprotein (fat-protein) fraction of the blood. In healthy adults in the United States, the total tocopherol content of the plasma ranges from 0.5 to 1.2 mg/100 ml. A level below 0.5 mg is a red flag. The predominant form of vitamin E in both the plasma and red cells is alpha tocopherol, which accounts for 83 percent of the total tocopherol; gamma tocopherol accounts for most of the remainder.

Vitamin E is stored in fatty tissue, the liver, and muscles primarily, although small amounts are stored in most body tissues. Relatively high amounts are found in the adrenal and pituitary glands, heart, lungs, testes, and uterus. There is little transfer of vitamin E across the placenta, so newborns have low tissue stores.

However, many researchers today believe we need 100 to 1,800 IU of vitamin E each day if we wish to prevent maladies, particularly those associated with coronary heart disease and aging.

Although clinical evidence of vitamin E deficiency that is ameliorated by vitamin E therapy has been observed in premature infants and in patients with malabsorption syndromes, research on the vitamin E requirement for healthy adults is still not conclusive.[5] Vitamin E requirements may vary more than fivefold, depending on dietary intake and/or tissue composition from previous dietary habits.

With the current emphasis on low-fat diets and substituting polyunsaturated fats for saturated, we may be depleting our vitamin E stores. The more polyunsaturated fatty acids you take in, the more the impact on your vitamin E status.[6]

Take the amount of vitamin E to prevent free-radical damage, for example. Breath pentane expiration is used as an index of oxidized fat in tissues. Daily intake of 1,000 IU vitamin E for ten days significantly reduced breath pentane output in healthy adults consuming a normal, mixed diet. On the basis of these study results, it is inferred that an undesirable chronic level of oxidized fat occurs in tissues and that vitamin E supplementation can decrease it.

Daniel Perry, executive director of Alliance for Aging Research, points out that fewer than 10 percent of Americans currently eat the five daily servings of fruits and vegetables recommended by the National Cancer Institute and other government health agencies. "It's irrelevant what the diet looks like in the case of vitamin E," adds Jeffrey Blumberg, Ph.D., chief of the Antioxidants Research Laboratory at Tufts University, Boston, Massachusetts. "You won't get 100 IU of vitamin E a day in dietary intake."[7]

The FDA, in response to the interest in vitamin E, issued the following official statement on September 23, 1971:

> "Vitamin E displays no known medical therapeutic effects. Articles have appeared in the medical literature claiming therapeutic benefits from the use of vitamin E beyond its value to prevent or correct a dietary deficiency. At present there is no unequivocal evidence that vitamin E has any therapeutic use.
>
> "Clinical use of vitamin E for many conditions has been reported without conclusive findings. Some of

these are habitual abortion, sterility, toxemias of pregnancy, lack of libido, aging, muscular dystrophy, muscle weakness, angina pectoris, coronary heart disease, leg cramps, peripheral vascular disease, and liver disease.

"The FDA is sympathetic to all who are affected by these conditions and joins those who wish vitamin E would be effective as claimed. Unfortunately, scientific studies do not back up these claims."

In 1990, the FDA described the "Vitamin of the Month" in its publication *FDA Consumer,* stating:

"Vitamin E is a fat-soluble vitamin not recognized as an essential nutrient until the 1960s, about forty years after its discovery....

"Vitamin E prevents potentially harmful oxidation of polyunsaturated fatty acids in the body, which would lead to cell damage; important in protecting red blood cell membranes from oxidation.

"Vitamin E deficiency can cause anemia as a result of red blood cell destruction and nerve damage. However, deficiency is rare and mainly occurs in premature, very low birth weight infants and people with fat-absorption disorders, such as cystic fibrosis."[8]

In 1997, however, everything is gradually changing, as you have read in this book. Experts in nutrition are slowly moving away from making recommended daily allowances that prevent just symptoms of deficiency to making allowances that take into consideration chronic diseases.[9]

PRECAUTIONS

If some substance has an effect on the human body, chances are it has the potential for an adverse effect. High intake of vitamin E by humans has generally been considered safe with few side effects, although some concerns about high intravenous doses of vitamin E for premature infants have been raised.[10] There have also been reports in the literature of high doses of vitamin E causing such conditions as creatinuria (signifying an impact on the kidneys) and fatigue, but these have not been reported in well-controlled studies.[11, 12] There have been some reports of gastrointestinal upsets.[13]

In double-blind studies of vitamin E even at doses as high as 3,200 IU for three weeks to six months, however, few side effects were noted. In a study of eighteen people who were given 3,200 IU of vitamin E for nine weeks, the only adverse symptoms recorded were intestinal cramps in one subject and diarrhea in three other subjects. Even over a long time—six years—healthy volunteers aged thirty-nine to fifty-six who were given either 3 mg or 100 mg daily of vitamin E capsules reported no adverse effects in either group for the entire period.[14] The same lack of adverse effects was also reported in diabetics receiving 2,000 IU vitamin E daily for six weeks.[15]

Two hundred college students received 600 IU dl-alpha tocopherol (synthetic vitamin E) or a placebo daily for twenty-eight days in one randomized, double-blind trial. There was no effect on work performance, sexuality, or general well-being. Subjects did not report muscular weakness or gastrointestinal disturbances. There was no effect on blood-clotting time, total white cell count, or creatine in the blood, which might show an effect on the kidneys. Serum triglycerides (blood fats) were elevated in women only. Serum thyroid hormone levels were reduced in this study, but a later study could not confirm this observation.[16]

No evidence of mutagenicity or birth defects or cancer has been reported.[17]

These studies do not prove that vitamin E is harmless for everyone and that you can take it without any problem. Vitamin E supplementation has been found to potentiate an increase in blood-clotting time in individuals with disease- or drug-induced vitamin K deficiency. Therefore, high levels of vitamin E are not advised during anticoagulant therapy.[18] Vitamin E has not been found to produce coagulation abnormalities in individuals who are not vitamin K deficient.[19] It has been recommended, however, that patients about to undergo major surgery avoid taking high levels of vitamin E for at least two weeks before to avoid the slim possibility of excess bleeding.

DO YOU NEED SUPPLEMENTS IF YOU ARE HEALTHY?

The Washington, D.C.–based Alliance for Aging Research, a scientific-advisory-panel, nongovernmental, nonprofit group working to advance medical research on human aging, advised healthy adults to sharply increase their intake of selected antioxidant nutrients.

The panel says adults should each day consume from 250 mg to 1,000 mg of vitamin C, from 100 IU to 400 IU of vitamin E, and from 10 mg to 30 mg of beta-carotene as a means of preventing chronic, age-related diseases.

Agencies including the FDA and the National Academy of Sciences, which advises the U.S. Department of Agriculture on changes in the recommended daily allowances for nutritional intake, say such a recommendation is premature.

The Alliance recommends intake levels four to sixteen times higher than the RDA. The RDA for vitamin C is 60 mg and 30 IU for vitamin E. None has been established for beta-carotene.

If you

- are under psychological stress
- live in a polluted environment
- exercise vigorously
- are on a low-fat diet with polyunsaturated fats
- take certain medications
- smoke
- drink alcohol
- have a history of heart disease
- have cancer in your family

vitamin E is a preventive. It can ameliorate certain conditions. It is not curative unless there is a deficiency.

There are also reports in the current scientific literature that the effects of vitamin E are enhanced if taken with zinc or tea.

How much do you, as an individual, need? If some researchers are correct, there will be more precise measurements to tell you.

Researchers at the University of Pennsylvania Medical Center have developed what they claim to be the first method to measure a nearly ubiquitous biochemical, easily detected in either blood or urine, that reflects the effect in the living body of those troublemakers, free radicals. The chemical being measured is 8-epi PGF2-alpha. It was used to determine the effects in smokers who either switched to nicotine patches or took aspirin or vitamins C and E.

"What this represents is a noninvasive, quantitative marker of a process that has been implicated in the origin of a wide repertoire of diseases, including cancer and heart disease," says senior author Garret A. FitzGerald, M.D., chairman of the department of pharmacology and a professor of cardiovascular medicine. "So, for the first time, we can develop a rational basis for attributing a role for free radicals in those diseases, for establishing antioxidant doses of vitamins or drugs, and, therefore, for testing those doses in relevant diseases."[20]

One result of the finding could be large-scale clinical trials to assess the efficacy of antioxidant vitamins and other compounds in preventing the damage caused by free radicals.[21]

"Our problem, up to now, has been that we have had very little information at all as to what might be an appropriate antioxidant dose or dosing interval of any particular vitamin or drug," says Dr. FitzGerald. "This has led to a certain amount of confusion among members of the public and in the medical literature. And the attraction of this test is that it's a specific, chemically stable marker of antioxidant activity that can be measured with great accuracy."

Additionally, the research provides a way to identify individuals with inadequate inborn defenses against free radicals, who might, therefore, benefit from antioxidant vitamin or drug interventions to prevent disabling or life-threatening diseases later in life.

"The imbalance between the generation of reactive free radicals and the body's antioxidant defenses is detectable by this approach in people who don't have any overt disease—in this case smokers," Dr. FitzGerald notes. "The same may be true as far as alcohol consumption and other risk factors are concerned, which raises the possibility that this test may give us a handle on the role of free radicals in the evolution of disease before it is clinically manifest."

The American Heart Association still maintains that you can get sufficient vitamin E from the diet.

"The amount of vitamin E given in this intervention study, and others, is far in excess of what can be obtained from the diet alone," William Pryor, Ph.D., director, Biodynamics Institute, Louisiana State University, noted, commenting on the American Heart Association's recognition of the antioxidant vitamin. He maintains, "Vitamin E has come of age, and we pioneers in the research of this exciting antioxidant are pleased to see that the American Heart Association is recognizing its significance. It's important that the public recognize it is impossible to get the amount of vitamin E from food that is being used in these human intervention trials. Therefore, it is necessary to take a vitamin E supplement."

Robert Russell, M.D., from Tufts University, noted that 100 to 200 IU of vitamin E is far in excess of the level that can be achieved in an otherwise healthful diet.[22] "Yet, the official American Heart Association position, reiterated in the December 18, 1996 release, persists in recommending that healthy people get adequate vitamin intakes from eating a variety of foods rather than from supplements."

Whether you should take supplemental vitamin E is up to you. As you have read in this book, the vitamin has preventive and therapeutic potential.

Elizabeth Yetley, Ph.D., acting director of the Office of Special Nutritionals at the Food and Drug Administration, was quoted in the *Journal of the American Medical Association* as saying that the issue of antioxidants' disease prevention potential is going to get "hotter before it gets resolved."

She referred to the existing data that are thorough enough to support the routine use of antioxidant vitamins and minerals to ward off such illnesses as cancer and cardiovascular disease that have been associated with oxidative cell damages.[23]

Vitamin E, the vitamin in search of a disease, the "shady lady" of research, has at last become the object of much scientific and public attention.

There is no doubt now that vitamin E is essential for your health. Beyond the amount to prevent deficiency lies the enigma. How much vitamin E can protect us from heart disease, cancer, and the other ills to which we are vulnerable?

In the meantime, it is wise, of course, to check with your physician before embarking on high doses of vitamin E. You might follow the lead of Dr. Myron Brin, formerly with Hoffmann–La Roche, who once said he took vitamin E just like "OBS" in bridge:

"When you are playing trump, you play an extra round to be sure all the trump has been thrown. It's called OBS, 'Oh, be sure!' Taking supplementary vitamin E is like that; it is insurance."

Dr. Vishwa Singh, the current director of human-nutrition research at Hoffmann–La Roche, says that "vitamin E is an important antioxidant. There is overwhelming evidence that it plays an important role in prevention of chronic diseases. The evidence is especially compelling regarding the risk of coronary heart disease. Not only are there the epidemiologic data, but there is correlation in animal data and early-intervention human trials data that vitamin E is useful in reducing the risk of coronary heart disease. The evidence is not yet as strong in the cancer area, but there are some very promising studies."

USDA/Tufts University's Dr. Blumberg says, when asked

whether one should take vitamin E and how much, "I tell people, 'Look at your diet...what you are eating....How healthful is it? What is your personal risk for heart disease? Eye disease? Did your parents or siblings have the disease?... When did they get it?'

"Your family history is a good indicator of your own risk. Then there are other issues...Do you smoke? Live in an urban environment? Vitamin E can protect against that kind of thing. The scientific literature says so."

The answer to whether you should take 100 to 400 IU of vitamin E depends upon your personal and environmental factors.

Does Dr. Blumberg take it?

Every day he takes 400 IU of vitamin E! So do most of the experts interviewed for this book. So does the author of this book.

12

VITAMIN E IN RAW, PROCESSED, AND COOKED FOOD

Vitamin E is so "hot" today because

- it is an antioxidant that helps prevent rancidity of fat.
- it is not toxic in large amounts.
- it is inexpensive.

Until the early nineties when a steady stream of studies began to suggest that vitamin E could offset some of the disabilities that accompany aging, vitamin E was not a hot property.

In recent years, however, such studies have boosted demand, increasing the market by more than 10 percent a year.[1] Archer Daniels Midland is one of the biggest suppliers of the raw vitamin, extracted from the distillate left over from the manufacture of soy and other vegetable oils; vitamin E sales in 1995 totaled over $500 million in the United States.

But which one to use?

There is natural vitamin E and synthetic vitamin E. Is there a difference?

In price, there certainly is. At retail prices, natural vitamin E is two to two and a half times as expensive. A bottle of one hundred capsules of 400 IU natural vitamin E costs $13 to $15 at this writing compared to $5.50 to $8.50 for the same quantity of synthetic vitamin E. Processing the vegetable oil distillate and encapsulation are more expensive than converting synthetic raw material into product. Scarcity of supply is also a factor in the higher prices for natural vitamin E, manufacturers contend.[2]

The term *vitamin E* covers eight compounds found in nature. Four of them are called tocopherols and four tocotrienols, and they are identified by the prefixes *alpha, beta, gamma,* and *delta.* Alpha tocopherol is the most common and biologically the most active of these naturally occurring forms of vitamin E.

The nature-made vitamin E is isolated from vegetable oils, primarily soy. Synthetic vitamin E is extracted from petrochemicals.

Nature-made vitamin E is d-alpha tocopherol and that's all.

Man-made vitamin E is dl-alpha tocopherol, a mixture of eight similar chemicals, only one of which is very similar to natural vitamin E. The other seven chemicals in the mixture have different makeups and lower biological activity. Natural-source vitamin E has a 36 percent greater potency than the synthetic, and in animal studies it has been reported to be almost twice as effective. In one respected study, the natural vitamin stayed in the tissue longer than the synthetic product.[3]

You can tell the natural supplement on a label because it begins with *d.* The synthetic with *dl.* The dl form of vitamin E is widely used as an antioxidant in stablizing edible oils and fats and fat-containing food products.

A spokesperson for a major producer of vitamin E says

that, as far as it is known, there is no difference between natural and synthetic vitamin E as it relates to the human body. Either one is fine. He said most food producers use synthetic vitamin E to fortify their products. But when the products are presented in IUs, both the natural and the synthetic are equal—400 IU of natural vitamin E and 400 IU of synthetic are equal.

Vitamin E has been one of the fastest-growing single-entity vitamins in the past two years. At the manufacturing level, sales of natural vitamin E jumped 40 percent in one year, indicating the market has almost doubled in three years.[4]

Worldwide refined vitamin E sales are roughly $1 billion—$400 million for animals, $150 million for food, $450 million for supplements, and $20 million for health and beauty care. The United States represents about half of this demand. One of the major processors of vitamin E, Archer Daniels Midland, of Decatur, Illinois, reports that growth of natural vitamin E is "limited by supply" and not by demand.

"We are selling everything we can make," a spokesperson for the company said.[5]

Leading suppliers of synthetics to the animal and human markets are Roche, BASF, Eisai, and Rhone-Poulenc.

Vitamin E is available in soft gelatin capsules, as chewable or effervescent tablets, or in ampoules and is found in most multivitamin supplements. It is usually measured and sold in international units, which are equivalent regardless of the source of vitamin E. While natural vitamin E is gram for gram 50 percent more active than synthetic vitamin E, 100 IU of natural vitamin E will offer the same activity as 100 IU of the synthesized version. You may also read *acetate* or *succinate* on the labels. These esters are added because alpha tocopherol loses potency when exposed to air, heat, and light. If the capsules of vitamin E acetate or succinate are stored in a cool, dark place, there is no stability problem. Alpha tocopherol supplements will retain potency for at least three years.[6]

The vitamin E acetate is also used in cosmetics and liquid vitamin drops because of its stability.

LABELING

Vitamin E content is generally expressed by biological activity, using the scale of international units (IU). By this system, 1 mg of d-alpha tocopherol, biologically the most active of the naturally occurring forms of vitamin E, is equivalent to 1.49 IU of vitamin E. The biological activity of 1 mg of dl-a-tocopherol acetate, the manufactured form of vitamin E commonly used in food enrichment, is equivalent to 1 IU.

Since 1992, instead of the familiar recommended daily allowances (RDAs) on food labels, producers have had to have recommended daily intakes (RDIs). FDA nutritionist John Wallingford, Ph.D., says the RDIs are just for labeling purposes. This is because the RDAs have specific recommendations based on age and sex and that would be too complex to put on a product label.

The conservatives in medicine and nutrition have loudly been proclaiming that vitamin E is widespread in nature and in food, and that therefore we all get more than enough vitamin E if we eat the normal American diet. However, new research with more sensitive instruments has shown a wide variation in the amount of active vitamin E in food, its availability to humans, and its fate when boiled, baked, fried, broiled, or frozen.

Like a voice crying in the wilderness, Robert Harris of the Massachusetts Institute of Technology in Cambridge, Massachusetts, maintained in 1962 that "the literature relating to the effects of storage and processing on the retention of tocopherols in foods is limited, controversial, and inadequate."

He pointed out that vitamin E activity of foods is always less—perhaps 40 percent less—than the total tocopherol content, and there is essentially no published data on the true vitamin E activity of individual foods, either raw or processed.

Professor Harris said that using the paper chromatography method of analysis, it was shown that wheat flour artificially "aged" and bleached with chlorine dioxide lost 80 percent of its tocopherols. Another study of Australian whole wheat bread showed that the bread's tocopherol dropped from 2.3 mg per million to 0.72 mg per million after chlorine dioxide bleaching.

Professor Harris further pointed out that the tocopherol content of food may rise or fall with ripeness. For instance, the spice paprika rose from 0.7 mg percent when half ripe to 4.3 mg percent when ripe. On the other hand, sunflower seeds decreased from 76 mg percent on the seventh day after blooming to 0.4 mg percent when ripe.

Professor Harris also found that after 30 minutes of heating at 175°C, coconut oil lost 21 percent of its tocopherol content, and after six months of storage at 37°C, it lost 26 percent; peanut oil lost 31 percent of its tocopherols after heating and 43 percent after storage; and sesame oil, 36 percent and 42 percent respectively.

Dr. David Herting and Emma-Jane Drury of Kodak Research Laboratories reported in the *Journal of Nutrition* a year later that their analysis of vegetable oils and fats from 11 different types of plants showed as low as zero mg of alpha tocopherol per gram in castor bean and linseed oils and as high as 1,276 mg per gram in wheat germ oil.

The two researchers found that in various types of vegetable oils and fats, the tocopherol levels appeared to be influenced by:

- source of the plant
- soil
- feed nutrients
- time of harvest
- weather
- stability after harvest
- refining procedure
- commercial hydrogenation (solidifying) procedures

Cow's milk, for example, can vary in its vitamin E content from 0.21 mg per quart in early spring to 1.5 mg per quart, which reflects not only the variation in the original grain but probably also differences in processing techniques.

Cooking oils may be high in tocopherols but not in *alpha tocopherol*—the most potent form for humans.

Destruction of vitamin E is accelerated not only by oxygen but by exposure to light, heat, alkali, and the presence of certain trace minerals such as iron and copper.[7]

The milling of grains removes about 80 percent of the vitamin E, for example, in converting whole wheat to white flour, and in processing corn, oats, and rice.

Various methods of processing cause considerable destruction of vitamin E. Here are some of the preservation and cooking methods that deplete vitamin E:

- Dehydration causes 36 to 45 percent loss of alpha tocopherol in chicken and beef, but little or none in pork.

- Canning causes losses of 41 to 65 percent of the alpha tocopherol content of meats and vegetables.
- Frozen storage will also degrade vitamin E.
- An 80 percent destruction occurs during the roasting of nuts.
- Flaking, shredding, puffing, and other procedures to process grain to produce cereals results in as much as a 90 percent loss of vitamin E.
- Deep-fat frying of foods causes vitamin E losses of 32 to 75 percent.

Dr. Bunnell said that the "typical diet" is a matter of controversy and not fact so that any selection of foods is a compromise. Nevertheless, he said, it was generally agreed that the principal source of vitamin E in the American diet is vegetable oils and fats.

He and his colleagues purchased all the different foods in local grocery stores and, in some instances, purchased several brands of one type of food. They emphasized the selection of foods processed in or containing vegetable oils.

The fresh foods were prepared and cooked, when possible, in the laboratory test kitchen. Frozen foods were prepared according to the directions on the package.

Dr. Bunnell and his group studied only the vitamin E losses involved in cooking of the food, not the losses involved in the commercial processing of food.

Milk averaged about 1.06 mg of tocopherol per quart in midfall. Evaporated milk contained 0.66 mg per quart, condensed milk 1.29, and nonfat dry milk 0.02 mg of tocopherol per quart.

They found that the vitamin E levels in both liquid and powdered imitation milks varied in E content from 3.46 to 6.8 mg per quart. They also found that human milk averaged

1.14 mg of alpha tocopherol per quart whether it was fresh, frozen, or pasteurized, lending further support to those who advocate breast-feeding of babies.

The vitamin E content of human milk, 2 to 5 IU in about a quart, is considered adequate for full-term infants. Cow's milk differs from human milk. It contains only one-tenth to one-half as much vitamin E, varying with what the cow eats. It is much lower in polyunsaturated fats, containing about half as much.[8] Increased vitamin E is required for both premature and full-term infants fed commercial formulas made from vegetable oils that are high in polyunsaturated fats. According to the Committee on Nutrition of the Academy of Pediatrics, full-term infants require at least 0.7 IU of vitamin E per gram of linoleic acid in a formula preparation.[9]

The richest natural sources of vitamin E are wheat germ, safflower, and sunflower oils, and nuts and whole grains. Smaller amounts are in foods like peaches and prunes. Foods of animal origins are generally low in vitamin E.

It is estimated that about 64 percent of vitamin E intake in our "normal" diet is supplied by salad oils, margarine, and shortening; about 11 percent by fruits and vegetables; and about 7 percent by grains and grain products.[10]

"Today," Dr. Bunnell wrote, "practically all the commercial deep-fat-fried frozen foods, such as french fried potatoes, scallops, shrimp, and chicken, are prepared in vegetable oils or shortening. Therefore, these foods should supply a significant amount of tocopherol in the diet. However, examination of the data reveals that this is not so.

The relatively low tocopherol content in a wide variety of such frozen foods prompted the investigation of the stability of tocopherol in foods fried in vegetable oils and placed in freezer storage. Frozen foods that had been fried in vegetable oils were surprisingly low in tocopherol, indicating a severe loss of tocopherol during freezer storage. Dr. Bunnell commented that the loss of tocopherol in frozen foods is of considerable importance currently because of the great amount of frozen food products consumed.

The tocopherol content of canned vegetables is low in comparison to fresh or frozen vegetables. Fresh peas, for example, contain .55 mg of tocopherol per gram; frozen, .25 mg; and canned, .09 mg.

Meat, fish, and poultry supply low to moderate amounts of tocopherol, with fish being the best apparent source. Salmon steak had the highest alpha tocopherol content among the fish assayed in the study.

Desserts, the group found, can vary considerably in alpha tocopherol content. Cookies and pies made with vegetable oil shortening may be a good source of tocopherol. Snack foods such as fresh potato chips cooked in fresh vegetable oil can also be rich in tocopherol.

The Hoffmann–La Roche researchers prepared typical breakfast, lunch, and dinner menus, which indicated a daily tocopherol intake ranging from 2.6 to 15.4 mg, with an overall average intake of 7.4 mg. This is about half the previous estimates of daily vitamin E intake and less than one-fourth of the minimum daily requirement set by the National Academy of Sciences.

More than 55 percent of the food we eat today is processed. A study done at the request of the federal government showed frozen TV dinners are deficient in vitamin E.

The evidence is mounting that the more processed foods we eat and the longer our food is stored, the less vitamin E we are ingesting. Ironically, more than 80 percent of the vitamin E distilled or manufactured in the United States today goes to enrich animal feed, not human food.

GOING IN THE WRONG DIRECTION?

The Food and Nutrition Board of the National Academy of Sciences sets the recommended daily allowances, which the FDA follows. The Food and Nutrition Board has recommended a reduction in the RDA for vitamin E from 30 IU to 15 IU. Why didn't the FDA lower the amount on food labels?

The FDA was prohibited from making changes in the specific vitamins for a period after the passage of the labeling act, so they used the 1976 RDAs. The RDIs (based on the 1976 RDAs) for the major antioxidant nutrients now on your food labels are:

- vitamin A, 5,000 IU
- vitamin E, 30 IU
- vitamin C, 60 mg

There is none for beta-carotene.

Whether the RDI for vitamin E will actually be reduced to 15 IU for adult men and 10 IU for adult women is still in dispute. When the Food and Nutrition Board proposed and published the reduction in the *Federal Register,* as required, many experts opposed the lowering of the standard. At this writing, an expert committee is in formation to reevaluate the RDIs for vitamin E and other antioxidants.

Dr. Jeffrey Blumberg, chief of the Antioxidants Research Laboratory at Tufts University, Boston, said, "It would be an enormous step backwards for public health if the RDI is rolled back to 15 IU.

"When they do that on food labeling, it affects the food composition. Instead of having thirty IU, food processors will say they have one hundred percent of RDI vitamin E added when they have fifteen IU.

"You can get thirty IU if you fortify breakfast cereals with more vitamins."

"There is a link between RDAs and health and preventing chronic diseases. While some media may have overhyped vitamin E as a magic pill, there is extraordinary, compelling evidence that vitamin E has a therapeutic use. Even the American Heart Association says so. It helps protect against heart disease and some forms of cancer."

He said it is not a conspiracy to cut back on the RDA for vitamin E, but it is "inappropriate and insensitive."

And as far as Dr. Blumberg is concerned, it's "very frustrating!"[11]

Not only do we have RDIs replacing RDAs on our food labels, we also have *daily reference values* (*DRVs*) for nutrients for which no set of standards previously existed, such as fat, cholesterol, carbohydrates, proteins, and fibers. DRVs are usually based on a two-thousand-calorie-per-day diet. This level was chosen because many health experts say it approximates the maintenance calorie requirement of the group most often targeted for weight reduction: postmenopausal women.

If you are confused, you are not the only one. Many among the experts in nutrition and food production as well as the public have had a hard time with the changes.

The bottom line is that most experts who are studying the effects of vitamin E in prevention and in chronic diseases believe it is difficult to obtain enough vitamin E in your food. There may, however, be benefits from obtaining vitamin E in food in combination with other nutrients.

A list of foods and the amount of vitamin E they contain is in Appendix I. So, with the advice of a qualified professional, you may want to take supplemental vitamin E.

GOOD SOURCES OF VITAMIN E

*The serving sizes contain—

+   *1–24 percent of the U.S. RDA for adults and children over 4*

++   *25–39 percent of the U.S. RDA for adults and children over 4*

+++ *40 percent or more of the U.S. RDA for adults and children over 4*

Food	Serving Size	% of RDA*

BREAD, CEREALS, AND OTHER GRAIN PRODUCTS

Food	Serving Size	% of RDA*
Multigrain cereals, cooked	2/3 cup	+
Ready-to-eat cereals, fortified	1 ounce	+++
Wheat germ, plain	2 tablespoons	++

FRUITS

Food	Serving Size	% of RDA*
Apple, baked, unsweetened	1 medium	+
Apricots, canned, juice-pack	1/2 cup	+
Nectarine, raw	1 medium	+
Peaches, canned, juice-pack	1/2 cup	+

VEGETABLES

Food	Serving Size	% of RDA*
Chard, cooked	1/2 cup	+
Dandelion greens, cooked	1/2 cup	+
Kohlrabi, cooked	1/2 cup	+

Mustard greens, cooked .... 1/2 cup +
Pumpkin, cooked .... 1/2 cup +
Turnip greens, cooked .... 1/2 cup +

MEAT, POULTRY, FISH, AND ALTERNATES

Meat and Poultry

Liver, chicken, or turkey,
  braised .... 1/2 cup diced +

Fish and Seafood

Clams; steamed, boiled, or
  canned; drained .... 3 ounces +
Croaker, mackerel, mullet,
  or ocean perch; baked
  or broiled .... 3 ounces +
Mackerel, canned, drained .... 3 ounces +
Salmon:
  Baked, broiled, steamed,
    or poached .... 3 ounces +
    canned, drained .... 3 ounces +
Scallops, baked or broiled .... 3 ounces +
Shrimp:
  Broiled, steamed, or
    boiled .... 3 ounces + +
    canned, drained .... 3 ounces +

Nuts and Seeds

Almonds, unroasted .... 2 tablespoons + + +
Brazil nuts .... 2 tablespoons +
Filberts (hazelnuts) .... 2 tablespoons + + +
Peanut butter .... 2 tablespoons + +
Peanuts, roasted or
  dry-roasted .... 2 tablespoons +
Sunflower seeds, hulled,
  roasted, or dry-roasted .... 2 tablespoons + + +

_____
U.S. Dept. of Agriculture

APPENDIX II

VITAMIN E CONTENT OF FOODS

Product	Total Tocopherol (mg %)	Alpha Tocopherol (mg %)	% Lipid	Alpha Tocopherol (mg/gm lipid)
MEATS				
Bacon (fried)	.59	.53	39.70	.001
Ham steak (fried)	.52	.28	6.80	.040
Pork sausage (fried)	.32	.16	35.00	.005
Liverwurst	.69	.35	27.00	.013
Bologna	.49	.06	26.60	.002
Salami	.68	.11	16.00	.007
Ground beef (panfried)	.63	.37	11.10	.033
Fresh beef liver (broiled)	1.62	.63	5.80	.110
Fresh veal cutlet (panfried)	.24	.05	1.60	.030
T-bone beefsteak (broiled)	.55	.13	9.50	.014
Lamb chops (broiled)	.32	.16	13.30	.012
Pork chops (panfried)	.60	.16	19.50	.008
FISH				
Fillet of haddock (broiled)	1.20	.60	.18	3.300
Salmon steak (broiled)	1.81	1.35	3.20	.420
Deep-fried frozen shrimp				
oven-heated	6.60	.60	12.90	.047
not heated	5.90	1.90	11.50	.165
Deep-fried frozen scallops				
oven-heated	6.20	.60	9.40	.064
not heated	3.90	.71	5.90	.120

POULTRY

Chicken breast (broiled)	.58	.37	3.90	.095
Frozen fried chicken				
Brand "A"				
oven-heated	.32	.04	23.80	.002
Brand "A-1" (same as "A" but bought at a different store)				
oven-heated	1.39	.38	20.00	.019
not heated	1.43	.40	19.00	.021
Brand "B"				
oven-heated	1.10	.16	18.00	.009
not heated	.80	.10	14.00	.007

VEGETABLES

Raw potato	.08	.05		
Baked potato	.05	.03		
Boiled potato	.06	.04		
Frozen french-fried potatoes				
Brand "A"				
oven-heated	.36	.12	6.80	.018
not heated	.64	.15	5.50	.270
Brand "B"				
oven-heated	1.59	.43	6.20	.069
not heated	1.22	.41	5.40	.076
Fresh yellow onion	.34	.22		
Frozen french-fried onion rings				
Brand "A"				
oven-heated	6.20	.72	25.60	.028
not heated	5.20	.60	20.60	.029
Brand "B"				
oven-heated	6.40	.65	23.20	.028
not heated	5.50	.52	17.20	.030
Baked beans,				
Boston style	1.16	.14		

Fresh peas	1.73	.55	1.74	.320
Canned green peas	.04	.02		
Frozen green peas				
cooked	.65	.25		
uncooked	.64	.22		
Canned green beans	.05	.03		
Frozen cut green beans				
cooked	.25	.11		
uncooked	.24	.09		
Canned leaf spinach	.06	.02		
Canned kernel corn	.09	.05		
Frozen kernel corn				
cooked	.48	.19		
uncooked	.49	.19		
Celery	.57	.38	.12	3.300
Carrots	.21	.11	.05	2.400
Lettuce	.17	.06	.11	.550
Fresh tomatoes	.85	.40	.07	5.400
Dry navy beans	1.68	.47	.60	.780
Cooked white rice	.27	.18	.50	.360

FRUITS AND FRUIT JUICES

Fresh strawberries	.29	.13	.13	1.020
Frozen sliced				
strawberries	.40	.21	.07	3.040
Fresh banana	.42	.22	.29	.760
Fresh cantaloupe	.31	.14	.20	.700
Fresh apple	.51	.31	.19	1.630
Canned tomato juice	.71	.22		
Canned grapefruit juice	.18	.04		
Fresh orange juice	.20	.04		

BREADS

White bread	.23	.10	2.60	.050
Whole-wheat bread	2.20	.45	2.80	.160

CEREALS

Oatmeal	3.23	2.27	6.33	.360
Corn flakes	.43	.12	.33	.360
Dry-processed rice cereal	.28	.04	.20	.200
Dry oat cereal	1.53	.60	2.30	.260
Yellow cornmeal	3.43	.64	3.80	.170
Hominy grits	1.17	.31	.90	.340
Processed wheat and barley cereal	2.45	.61	.98	.620

DESSERTS

Chocolate ice cream				
Brand "A"	1.02	.36	12.20	.030
Brand "B"	1.10	.37	10.70	.035
Vanilla ice cream	.39	.06	13.20	.005
Fresh-baked apple pie	15.70	2.50	10.60	.240
Fresh-baked blueberry pie	17.70	3.12	14.70	.210

Reprinted with permission of Hoffmann–La Roche and the *American Journal of Clinical Nutrition* from the article "Alpha Tocopherol Content of Foods," R. H. Bunnell, J. Keating, A. Quaresimo, and G. K. Parman, *American Journal of Clinical Nutrition* 17 (July 1965).

VITAMIN E IN EDIBLE PORTIONS OF FOOD

	Svg		Wt (g)	Cal	Vit E Alpha-Toc Eq
BAKED GOODS					
Apple dumpling	1	ea	151.00	357.00	3.240
Baklava	1	pce	78.00	333.00	1.990
Biscuit, whole wheat	1	ea	63.00	201.00	.980
Bread:					
Banana, recipe, w/margarine	1	pce	50.00	163.00	.650
Coffee, Spanish	1	ea	85.00	292.00	1.080
Cornbread, f/mix, prepared	1	pce	60.00	188.00	.720
Cornbread, rec, w/whole milk	1	pce	65.00	176.00	.650
Indian fry/Navajo	1	pce	90.00	296.00	1.260
Pita, 100% whole wheat, tstd	1	ea	41.00	120.00	.426
Pumpernickel	1	pce	32.00	80.00	.544
toasted	1	pce	29.00	79.80	.542
Pumpkin, recipe	1	pce	60.00	199.00	1.200
Rice, toasted	1	pce	23.00	81.40	1.360
Rice bran	1	pce	27.00	65.60	.432
toasted	1	pce	25.00	66.00	.675
Whole wheat, recipe	1	pce	23.00	63.90	.230
toasted	1	pce	42.00	128.00	.420

	Svg		Wt (g)	Cal	Vit E Alpha-Toc Eq
Baked Goods, continued					
Whole wheat, toasted	1	pce	29.00	80.30	.290
Bread stuffing/dressing:					
Cornbread, f/mix	.5	c	100.00	179.00	1.200
Plain, f/mix	1	c	140.00	249.00	1.960
Recipe	1	c	203.00	341.00	2.440
Brownies:					
w/nuts, commercial	1	ea	56.00	227.00	1.060
w/nuts, f/mix	1	ea	33.00	140.00	.660
w/walnuts, recipe	1	ea	20.00	93.20	.580
Cakes:					
Applesauce, w/o icing	1	pce	87.00	313.00	1.150
Banana, w/o icing	1	pce	87.00	245.00	1.300
Carrot, mix, w/o icing	1	pce	58.00	198.00	1.390
Carrot, w/crm chse icing, rec	1	pce	112.00	488.00	5.600
Cheesecake:	1	pce	92.00	295.00	1.750
Chocolate	1	pce	128.00	501.00	2.310
f/no-bake mix	1	pce	103.00	282.00	1.130
Recipe	1	pce	128.00	457.00	2.940
Recipe, w/cherry topping	1	pce	142.00	402.00	2.270
Chocolate:					
German, f/mix, w/icing	1	pce	111.00	404.00	2.220
Pudding type, f/mix	1	pce	77.00	270.00	2.310
Recipe, no frosting	1	pce	95.00	340.00	1.430
w/chocolate icing	1	pce	69.00	253.00	1.170
Coffee, recipe cinnamon+ crumb topping	1	pce	60.00	240.00	1.500
Coffee, f/mix	1	pce	72.00	229.00	1.300
Fruitcake, recipe	1	pce	84.00	302.00	2.100
Gingerbread, f/mix	1	pce	63.00	195.00	.945
Gingerbread, recipe	1	pce	110.00	392.00	2.640
Lemon, w/icing	1	pce	109.00	388.00	2.090
Oatmeal, w/icing	1	pce	110.00	410.00	1.560

	Svg		Wt (g)	Cal	Vit E Alpha-Toc Eq
Baked Goods, continued					
Pineapple upside-down, rec	1	pce	115.00	367.00	2.070
Poppyseed, w/o icing	1	pce	90.00	354.00	1.030
Pound:					
Commercial, not all butter	1	pce	30.00	117.00	.810
Old-fashion, w/margarine	1	pce	53.00	230.00	1.960
Recipe, w/margarine	1	pce	54.00	206.00	1.350
Shortcake, biscuit type, rec	1	ea	65.00	225.00	1.300
Spice, w/icing	1	pce	109.00	374.00	2.200
Sponge, chocolate, w/o icing	1	pce	66.00	195.00	.701
White:					
f/mix	1	pce	62.00	190.00	.992
f/mix, pudding type	1	pce	69.00	244.00	2.070
w/white frosting	1	pce	71.00	266.00	1.280
Yellow:					
f/mix	1	pce	69.00	221.00	1.240
f/mix, pudding type	1	pce	73.00	257.00	2.190
Recipe, no icing	1	pce	68.00	246.00	1.360
w/choc icing, commercial	1	pce	69.00	262.00	1.380
w/vanilla icing	1	pce	121.00	451.00	2.300
Cobbler:					
Apple	1	pce	104.00	199.00	.989
Cherry	1	pce	129.00	198.00	1.070
Peach	1	pce	130.00	205.00	2.200
Cookies:					
Butterscotch	1	ea	34.00	149.00	.957
Chocolate chip:					
Dietetic	1	ea	5.00	24.90	.129
f/mix	1	ea	16.00	79.40	.416
Recipe, w/margarine	4	ea	40.00	195.00	1.160
Chocolate:					
Sandwich, creme-filled	4	ea	40.00	189.00	.680
Sandwich, w/choc icing	1	ea	17.00	81.80	.340

	Svg		Wt (g)	Cal	Vit E Alpha-Toc Eq
Baked Goods, continued					
Sandwich, w/extra creme	1	ea	13.00	65.00	.416
Wafer	2	ea	12.00	52.00	.276
Fig Bar	4	ea	56.00	195.00	.672
Fortune	1	ea	8.00	30.20	.083
Gingersnap	1	ea	7.00	29.10	.196
Ladyfinger	4	ea	44.00	161.00	.572
Lemon bar	1	ea	16.00	69.50	.500
Marshmallow, choc-coated	1	ea	13.00	54.70	.390
Oatmeal, recipe	1	ea	15.00	67.10	.405
Oatmeal, refrig dough, baked	1	ea	12.00	56.50	.360
Pastry, apple, dietetic	1	ea	24.00	115.00	1.540
Peanut butter:					
Commercial	1	ea	15.00	71.60	.570
Recipe	4	ea	48.00	228.00	1.820
Refrigerated dough, baked	1	ea	12.00	60.40	.480
Pecan shortbread	1	ea	14.00	75.90	.532
Raisin, soft type	1	ea	15.00	60.20	.450
Sandwich-type, dietetic	1	ea	11.00	50.30	.440
Shortbread, commercial	4	ea	32.00	161.00	.928
Shortbread, recipe, w/marg	1	ea	11.00	60.10	.550
Sugar:					
Dietetic	1	ea	6.00	27.80	.192
Recipe, w/margarine	1	ea	14.00	66.10	.518
Refrigerated dough, bdk	4	ea	48.00	232.00	1.440
Whole wheat fruit & nut	1	ea	14.00	60.30	.403
Crackers:					
Club/Waverly	2	ea	8.00	40.20	.280
Ritz	10	ea	30.00	151.00	1.050
Rye	2	ea	14.00	46.80	.140
Rye, seasoned	1	ea	22.00	83.80	.440
Sesame seed	4	ea	12.00	60.20	.420
Wasa Rye Crisp	2	pce	17.00	58.50	.321

	Svg		Wt (g)	Cal	Vit E Alpha-Toc Eq
Baked Goods, continued					
Whole wheat, 100%	3	ea	12.00	48.10	.442
Whole wheat & bran	3	ea	12.00	48.00	.440
Cream puff, custard-filled	1	ea	110.00	284.00	1.580
Crepe, 7"	1	ea	50.00	117.00	.702
Danish pastry:					
Cheese	1	ea	71.00	266.00	1.990
Cinnamon	1	ea	88.00	355.00	2.460
Lemon or raspberry	1	ea	71.00	263.00	1.990
Doughnut:					
Cake:	1	ea	50.00	211.00	.500
Chocolate-iced	1	ea	43.00	204.00	.645
Sugared/glazed	1	ea	45.00	192.00	.450
Chocolate, w/choc icing	1	ea	71.00	273.00	2.170
Custard-filled, w/icing	1	ea	70.00	261.00	1.910
Eggless, carob-coated, raised	1	ea	78.00	285.00	2.750
Oriental	1	ea	18.00	75.30	.345
Wheat, sugared/glazed	1	ea	45.00	162.00	1.350
Eclair, chocolate, custard-filled	1	ea	94.00	246.00	1.790
French toast, rec, w/2% milk	1	pce	65.00	149.00	.715
Muffins:					
Blueberry:					
Commercial	1	ea	57.00	158.00	.570
f/mix	1	ea	45.00	135.00	.630
Recipe, w/2% milk	1	ea	57.00	163.00	.969
Buckwheat	1	ea	47.00	144.00	.596
Carrot	1	ea	58.00	177.00	.606
Chocolate chip	1	ea	58.00	190.00	.646
Cornmeal:					
Commercial	1	ea	57.00	174.00	.684
f/mix	1	ea	45.00	145.00	.675
Recipe, w/2% milk	1	ea	57.00	180.00	1.030
English, whole wheat, tstd	1	ea	50.00	111.00	.528

	Svg		Wt (g)	Cal	Vit E Alpha-Toc Eq

Baked Goods, continued

Fruit &/or nuts	1	ea	58.00	164.00	.610
Oat bran 2 5/8" dia	1	ea	47.00	127.00	.708
Plain, recipe, w/2% milk	1	ea	57.00	169.00	1.030
Plain, recipe, w/whole milk	1	ea	45.00	136.00	.810
Pumpkin, w/raisins	1	ea	58.00	181.00	.586
Wheat bran, from mix	1	ea	45.00	124.00	.675
Wheat bran, rec, w/2% milk	1	ea	57.00	161.00	1.310
Whole wheat	1	ea	47.00	142.00	.703
Zucchini	1	ea	58.00	210.00	.844

Pancakes:

Blueberry, recipe	1	ea	38.00	84.40	.570
Buckwheat, incomplete, f/mix	1	ea	27.00	56.20	.270
Buttermilk, recipe	1	ea	38.00	86.30	.532
Incomplete, f/mix	1	ea	38.00	82.80	.418
Plain, recipe	1	ea	27.00	61.30	.378
Rye	1	ea	21.00	62.60	.255

Pies, 1 piece = 1/8 of 9" pie, unless otherwise indicated:

Apple, frozen, baked	1	pce	125.00	296.00	2.000
Apple, recipe	1	pce	155.00	411.00	2.950
Banana cream, recipe	1	pce	148.00	398.00	2.520
Blackberry, recipe	1	pce	150.00	401.00	2.270
Blueberry, recipe	1	pce	147.00	360.00	3.090
Cherry, frozen, baked	1	pce	125.00	325.00	2.130
Cherry, recipe	1	pce	180.00	486.00	3.420
Chocolate cream	1	pce	142.00	400.00	2.270
Lemon meringue, recipe	1	pce	127.00	362.00	2.290
Peach, recipe	1	pce	139.00	375.00	3.280
Pecan, recipe	1	pce	122.00	503.00	2.320
Pumpkin, recipe	1	pce	155.00	316.00	2.170

Pop Tarts:

Brown sugar & cinnamon	1	ea	50.00	206.00	1.500
Fruit filled	1	ea	52.00	204.00	1.140

	Svg		Wt (g)	Cal	Vit E Alpha-Toc Eq
Baked Goods, continued					
Fruit filled	1	ea	54.00	212.00	1.190
Rolls:					
Cinnamon raisin nut, recipe	1	ea	57.00	196.00	.912
Dinner, commercial	1	ea	28.40	85.10	.284
Dinner, egg	1	ea	35.00	108.00	.350
Mexican swt, crumb topping	1	ea	79.00	291.00	1.350
Refrig dough, cinn, frosted	1	ea	30.00	109.00	.480
Scone:	1	ea	42.00	150.00	.895
Whole wheat	1	ea	42.00	145.00	1.070
Strudels:					
Apple	1	pce	71.00	195.00	1.420
Berry	1	pce	64.00	159.00	1.040
Cheese	1	pce	64.00	195.00	.690
Cherry	1	pce	64.00	179.00	.698
Toaster muffins:					
Blueberry	1	ea	33.00	103.00	.495
toasted	1	ea	31.00	103.00	.496
Cornmeal	1	ea	33.00	114.00	.528
toasted	1	ea	31.00	114.00	.496
Wheat bran & raisin	1	ea	36.00	106.00	.576
toasted	1	ea	34.00	106.00	.544
Turnover:					
Apple	1	ea	82.00	289.00	1.380
Berry	1	ea	78.00	277.00	1.510
Cherry	1	ea	78.00	238.00	1.090
Lemon	1	ea	78.00	238.00	1.160
Waffles:					
100% whole wheat/whl grain	1	ea	39.00	107.00	.531
Blueberry, 7", round	1	ea	75.00	186.00	.893
Buttermilk, recipe	1	ea	75.00	217.00	1.500
Complete, f/mix	1	ea	75.00	218.00	1.500
Cornmeal, 7", round	1	ea	75.00	209.00	1.410

	Svg		Wt (g)	Cal	Vit E Alpha-Toc Eq
Baked Goods, continued					
Frozen, toasted	1	ea	35.00	92.40	.455
Oat bran	1	ea	38.00	107.00	.573
Plain, recipe	1	ea	75.00	218.00	1.730
Wheat/bran/mixed grain	1	ea	38.00	116.00	.934

CHIPS & SNACKS

	Svg		Wt (g)	Cal	Vit E Alpha-Toc Eq
Plaintain chips	32	pce	34.60	180.00	1.870
Popcorn, microwave, lowfat, low sodium	1	c	5.80	23.80	.060
Potato chips, sour cream+onion	1	oz	28.40	151.00	1.320
Potato skins, white, chips	10	pce	20.00	112.00	.976

DAIRY & DAIRY PRODUCTS

	Svg		Wt (g)	Cal	Vit E Alpha-Toc Eq
Cream, heavy, whipped	2	c	238.00	821.00	2.380
Milk (other), soy	1	c	244.00	150.00	2.560
Milk beverages, instant breakfast:					
w/nonfat milk	1	c	282.00	216.00	5.300
w/1% milk	1	c	281.00	233.00	5.360
w/2% milk	1	c	281.00	252.00	5.410
w/whole milk	1	c	281.00	280.00	5.510
Ice crm bar/stick, cake-covered	1	ea	59.00	162.00	.768

EGGS

	Svg		Wt (g)	Cal	Vit E Alpha-Toc Eq
Deviled	1	ea	31.00	62.50	.858
Fried, whole in margarine	1	ea	46.00	91.50	.754
Scrambled:					
Fast food	1	ea	94.00	199.00	1.600
f/cholesterol-free frozen mix	1	c	153.00	278.00	3.670
f/dry eggs	1	c	214.00	475.00	6.270
f/powdered mixture	1	c	188.00	362.00	4.090

	Svg		Wt (g)	Cal	Vit E Alpha-Toc Eq
Eggs, continued					
w/milk+margarine	1	ea	61.00	101.00	.793
Yolk, cooked	1	ea	16.60	59.20	.494

FATS, OILS & SALAD DRESSINGS

	Svg		Wt (g)	Cal	Vit E Alpha-Toc Eq
Butter	1	c	227.00	1627.00	3.590
Butter, whipped	.5	c	75.60	542.00	1.190
Fats:					
Bacon grease/					
meat fat drippings	1	T	14.00	125.00	.310
Beef tallow, mono+diglycerides	1	T	12.80	109.00	.358
Beef tallow/drippings	1	c	205.00	1849.00	5.540
Chicken, rendered	1	c	205.00	1845.00	5.600
Pork lard	1	c	205.00	1849.00	2.460
Turkey (rendered)	1	c	205.00	1845.00	5.880
Margarine:					
corn oil/butter blend	1	T	14.20	102.00	1.600
Hard:					
Coconut+safflower+palm	.5	c	113.00	815.00	10.200
Hydrog soybn+cottonseed	.5	c	113.00	815.00	15.700
Stick, soybn+hydrog soybn	1	T	14.20	102.00	1.820
Imitation, 40% fat, hydrog soybn	1	tsp	4.80	21.10	.408
Soft:					
Hydrog soybn+cottonseed	1	c	227.00	1625.00	31.100
Hydrog soybn+hydrog palm	1	c	227.00	1625.00	18.200
Hydrog soybean+safflower	1	c	227.00	1625.00	27.200
Tub	1	c	227.00	1625.00	29.500
Spread, tub, hydrogenated					
soybean+cottonseed	1	c	229.00	1236.00	31.400
Mayonnaise:					
Imitation	1	T	15.00	34.80	.965
Imitation, soybean, no chol	1	T	14.00	67.50	.700
Low calorie	1	T	15.60	36.20	1.000

	Svg		Wt (g)	Cal	Vit E Alpha-Toc Eq
Fats, Oils & Salad Dressings, continued					
Low calorie/diet, low sodium	1	T	14.00	32.30	.532
Safflower+soybean	1	c	220.00	1577.00	48.400
Soybean	1	T	13.80	99.00	3.670
Oils:					
Almond	1	c	218.00	1927.00	85.600
Butter/ghee	1	c	205.00	1795.00	5.740
Canola	1	c	218.00	1927.00	50.100
Cocoa butter	1	c	218.00	1927.00	3.920
Cod liver	1	T	13.60	123.00	2.990
Corn	1	c	218.00	1927.00	46.000
Corn, mono+diglycerides	1	T	13.60	116.00	2.350
Cottonseed	1	c	218.00	1927.00	83.400
Cottonseed, mono+diglycerides	1	T	13.60	116.00	5.820
Hazelnut	1	c	218.00	1927.00	103.000
Herring	1	T	13.60	123.00	1.250
Linseed	1	T	13.60	120.00	.286
Mustard	1	T	14.00	124.00	1.460
Oat	1	T	13.60	120.00	1.960
Olive	1	c	216.00	1909.00	25.900
Palm	1	c	218.00	1927.00	47.600
Palm kernel	1	c	218.00	1879.00	8.280
Palm, mono+diglycerides	1	T	13.60	116.00	4.500
Palm, refined	1	T	13.60	121.00	2.970
Peanut	1	c	216.00	1909.00	27.900
Poppyseed	1	c	218.00	1927.00	24.900
Rice bran	1	c	218.00	1927.00	79.600
Safflower, linoleic >70%	1	c	218.00	1927.00	75.000
Salmon	1	T	13.60	123.00	2.600
Sardine	1	T	13.60	123.00	1.630
Sesame	1	c	218.00	1927.00	8.870
Soybean:	1	c	218.00	1927.00	37.600
Hydrogenated	1	T	14.20	126.00	2.320

	Svg		Wt (g)	Cal	Vit E Alpha-Toc Eq
Fats, Oils & Salad Dressings, continued					
Hydrogenated+cottonseed	1	c	218.00	1927.00	26.400
Hydrog/mono/diglycerides	1	T	13.60	116.00	2.220
Lecithin	1	T	13.60	104.00	2.370
Mono+diglycerides	1	T	13.60	116.00	2.220
Sunflower	1	c	218.00	1927.00	131.000
Walnut	1	c	218.00	1927.00	7.020
Wheat germ	1	T	13.60	120.00	24.900
Salad dressings:					
Bacon + tomato, low calorie	1	T	16.20	32.40	.648
Blue cheese/Roquefort	1	c	245.00	1234.00	22.800
Buttermilk, creamy	1	T	14.70	71.40	1.580
Caesar	.5	c	92.00	418.00	5.400
Cooked, recipe	1	T	16.00	25.10	.304
Creamy, reduced calorie	1	T	15.00	24.00	.285
Dijon Vinaigrette Lite	1	T	15.00	15.80	.225
French:	1	c	250.00	1075.00	21.100
Low calorie	1	c	260.00	348.00	3.900
Recipe	2	T	28.00	177.00	3.360
Honey mustard	1	T	15.60	50.40	.219
Italian	1	c	235.00	1097.00	20.200
Diet	1	T	15.00	15.80	.225
Italian (Seven Seas Viva)	1	T	15.00	70.10	1.290
Miracle Whip	1	c	235.00	917.00	9.400
Light	1	T	14.00	36.40	.602
Ranch	.5	c	119.00	436.00	4.760
Russian	1	c	245.00	1210.00	25.000
Sesame seed	2	T	30.60	136.00	1.530
Thousand island	1	c	250.00	943.00	10.000
Low calorie	1	c	245.00	390.00	18.600
Vinegar+oil, recipe	1	T	16.00	71.80	1.440
Vinaigrette	1	T	14.70	68.70	1.260

	Svg	Wt (g)	Cal	Vit E Alpha-Toc Eq
Fats, Oils & Salad Dressings, continued				
Shortening:				
Frying, hvy duty, hydrog palm	1 T	12.80	113.00	2.560
Hydrogenated soybean+				
hydrogenated cottonseed	1 T	12.80	113.00	1.150
Regular, lard+vegetable oil	1 T	12.80	115.00	1.880
Vegetable, hydrogenated soybean+				
cottonseed	1 c	205.00	1812.00	30.100

FRUITS & FRUIT JUICES

	Svg	Wt (g)	Cal	Vit E Alpha-Toc Eq
Apricots, dried halves	1 c	130.00	309.00	2.470
Avocado, California, mashed	.5 c	115.00	204.00	1.730
Avocado, cubes	1 c	150.00	242.00	3.410
Banana, dehydrated	1 c	100.00	346.00	1.020
Banana, green, fried	1 ea	90.00	158.00	2.010
Blueberries:				
Canned, w/heavy syrup	1 c	256.00	225.00	2.560
Fresh	1 c	145.00	81.20	1.450
Frozen, sweetened, thawed	1 c	230.00	186.00	2.300
Currant, black	1 c	112.00	70.60	1.130
Guava	1 ea	90.00	45.90	1.010
Kiwi fruit	1 ea	76.00	46.40	.851
Mango	1 ea	207.00	135.00	2.340
Mango, slices	1 c	165.00	107.00	1.870
Papaya:	1 ea	304.00	119.00	3.410
Sliced	1 c	140.00	54.60	1.570
Dried	1 pce	23.00	59.40	1.710
Peach halves, dried	10 ea	130.00	311.00	1.770
Pear halves, dried	10 ea	175.00	459.00	1.860
Plantain, fried (plantano maduro)	1 c	169.00	432.00	1.920
Plantain, green, fried (tostones)	1 c	111.00	264.00	3.000
Prunes, dried	10 ea	84.00	201.00	1.120

	Svg		Wt (g)	Cal	Vit E Alpha-Toc Eq
Fruits & Fruit Juices, continued					
Raisins, packed	1	c	165.00	488.00	2.200
Raisins, unpacked	1	c	145.00	429.00	1.930

GRAINS & GRAIN PRODUCTS

	Svg		Wt (g)	Cal	Vit E Alpha-Toc Eq
Barley, whole, dry	1	c	184.00	651.00	2.360
Buckwheat, w/outside skin	1	c	170.00	583.00	2.380
Buckwheat flour, whole groat	1	c	98.00	328.00	1.030
Cereals, cold (ready to eat):					
100% Bran	1	c	66.00	178.00	1.530
All-Bran	.33	c	28.40	70.70	.659
Amaranth flakes	1	c	38.00	134.00	3.220
Bran Chex	1	c	49.00	156.00	.564
Bran Flakes	1	c	39.00	127.00	.449
Bran Flakes, Post	1	c	47.00	152.00	.541
Cinnamon Toast Crunch	1	c	38.00	161.00	.513
Complete Bran	1	c	61.00	195.00	10.600
Corn Bran	1	c	36.00	125.00	.835
Corn Total	1	c	33.00	126.00	34.900
Cracklin' Oat Bran	1	c	60.00	229.00	.690
Crispy Wheat 'n Raisins	1	c	43.00	150.00	11.400
Fruit & Fibre, date+rsn+nut	.5	c	28.40	96.30	.659
Granola:					
Lowfat	1	c	111.00	422.00	17.100
Nature Valley	1	c	113.00	503.00	3.390
Recipe, w/oat+wheat germ	1	c	122.00	594.00	5.720
Honey Bran	1	c	35.00	119.00	.812
Honey Buckwheat Crisp	.75	c	28.40	110.00	6.710
King Vitamin	1	c	21.00	85.30	6.660
Most	1	c	52.00	175.00	55.000
Mueslix Five Grain Muesli	1	c	82.00	279.00	8.940
Multi-grain, cooked	1	c	246.00	200.00	3.420
Nutri Grain Corn	1	c	42.00	160.00	11.100

	Svg		Wt (g)	Cal	Vit E Alpha-Toc Eq
Grains & Grain Products, continued					
Nutri Grain Wheat	1	c	44.00	158.00	11.600
Product 19	1	c	33.00	126.00	34.900
Raisin Bran	1	c	56.00	175.00	1.300
Raisin Bran, Post	1	c	56.00	172.00	1.300
Raisin Bran, Total	1	c	52.00	162.00	1.210
Raisin Nut Bran	1	c	57.00	221.00	1.320
Total, wheat, w/calcium	1	c	33.00	116.00	34.900
Uncle Sam's High Fiber	1	c	110.00	427.00	1.580
Oat bran, dry	1	c	94.00	231.00	1.190
Oat grain, dry	1	c	156.00	607.00	1.950
Oats, rolled, baked value	1	c	80.00	307.00	.912
Oats, rolled, dry	1	c	81.00	311.00	.923
Quinoa, grain, dry	1	c	170.00	636.00	8.280
Rice, fried, meatless	1	c	166.00	264.00	2.460
Rice flour, dark	1	c	128.00	415.00	3.420
Rice flour, light	1	c	102.00	374.00	1.590
Rice grain	1	c	158.00	529.00	3.030
Rich polishings	1	c	105.00	278.00	6.350
Tortilla, flour, 8"	1	ea	35.40	115.00	.581
Tortilla, whole wheat	1	ea	35.00	73.20	.431
Wheat bran, baked value	.5	c	18.00	38.90	.470
Wheat bran, crude	.5	c	30.00	64.80	.783
Wheat germ:					
Crude	1	c	100.00	360.00	18.000
Baked value	1	c	75.00	270.00	13.500
Toasted	1	c	113.00	432.00	22.400
Wheat grain:					
Durum	.5	c	96.00	325.00	1.390
Hard white	.5	c	96.00	328.00	1.710
Soft white	.5	c	84.00	286.00	1.740
Whole:					
Hard red spring	.5	c	96.00	316.00	1.920

	Svg		Wt (g)	Cal	Vit E Alpha-Toc Eq
Grains & Grain Products, continued					
Hard red winter, dry	.5	c	96.00	314.00	1.560
Soft red winter	.5	c	84.00	278.00	1.340

MEATS: FISH & SHELLFISH

	Svg		Wt (g)	Cal	Vit E Alpha-Toc Eq
Abalone:					
Canned	5.29	oz	150.00	120.00	7.500
Fried	2	oz	56.70	107.00	3.020
Steamed/poached	5.29	oz	150.00	315.00	12.000
Anchovy, cnd, oil pack, drnd	5	ea	20.00	42.00	1.000
Anchovy, cooked	10	ea	40.00	84.00	2.000
Bass, saltwater, baked/brld	1	ea	101.00	125.00	2.770
Bass, striped, baked/broiled	2	oz	56.70	70.30	.680
Carp, baked/broiled	1	ea	170.00	275.00	4.660
Carp, floured/breaded, fried	4.66	oz	132.00	366.00	2.130
Catfish, brd/battered, baked	4.66	oz	132.00	399.00	4.200
Catfish, steamed/poached	4.66	oz	132.00	223.00	1.980
Caviar, black/red, granular	2	T	32.00	80.60	2.240
Clams:					
Baked/broiled, large	5	ea	150.00	209.00	3.160
Breaded, fried	5.29	oz	150.00	303.00	4.050
Cake/patty	1	ea	120.00	429.00	2.570
Canned, drained	5.64	oz	160.00	237.00	3.200
Smoked, oil pack	10	ea	100.00	175.00	1.970
Crab:					
Baked/broiled	4.16	oz	118.00	162.00	1.990
Blue:					
Canned	4.76	oz	135.00	134.00	1.350
Steamed/boiled	4.16	oz	118.00	120.00	1.180
Deviled	6.17	oz	175.00	342.00	3.820
Soft shell, floured/brd, fried	1	ea	65.00	217.00	1.630
Eel, baked/broiled	1	ea	159.00	375.00	7.950
Eel, steamed/poached	4.66	oz	132.00	304.00	6.600

	Svg		Wt (g)	Cal	Vit E Alpha-Toc Eq
Meats: Fish & Shellfish, continued					
Haddock, cake/patty	1	ea	120.00	239.00	1.210
Haddock, floured/brd, fried	1	ea	81.00	190.00	1.120
Halibut, Greenland, fillet, baked/broiled	.5	pce	159.00	380.00	7.000
Herring:					
Atlantic:					
Baked/broiled	1	ea	143.00	290.00	2.090
Pickled	4.94	oz	140.00	367.00	1.400
Smoked, kippered	1	ea	40.00	86.80	.400
Pacific , baked/broiled	1	ea	144.00	360.00	3.310
Lobster:					
Baked/broiled, diced	5.11	oz	145.00	168.00	1.470
Batter fried	5.11	oz	145.00	306.00	2.500
Tail, baked/broiled	1	ea	125.00	145.00	1.270
w/butter sauce	6.63	oz	188.00	448.00	2.130
Mackerel:					
Baked/broiled	2	oz	56.70	114.00	1.270
Cake/patty	1	ea	120.00	298.00	2.180
Jack, canned, drained	6.7	oz	190.00	296.00	2.660
Mussels, blue, steamed/bld	5.29	oz	150.00	258.00	2.220
Oysters:					
Eastern:					
Boiled/steamed	6	ea	42.00	57.50	.672
Breaded, fried	4.62	oz	131.00	258.00	2.990
Wild, baked/broiled	6.07	oz	172.00	124.00	2.670
Pacific, boiled/steamed	1	ea	38.00	61.90	.608
Salmon:					
Atlantic, wild, baked/broiled	.5	ea	154.00	280.00	2.930
Chinook, baked/broiled	3	oz	85.00	196.00	.867
Chinook, smoked/lox	2	oz	56.70	66.30	.766
Coho:					
Farmed, ckd, dry heat	1	ea	143.00	255.00	3.920

	Svg		Wt (g)	Cal	Vit E Alpha-Toc Eq

Meats: Fish & Shellfish, continued

	Svg		Wt (g)	Cal	Vit E Alpha-Toc Eq
Steamed/poached	.5	ea	155.00	285.00	1.550
Wild, cooked, dry heat	.5	ea	178.00	247.00	4.770
Pink, w/bone, cnd, not drnd	5.29	oz	150.00	209.00	2.100
Sockeye/red, baked/broiled	1	ea	155.00	335.00	3.880
Sockeye/red, canned, drained, unsalted	1	ea	369.00	565.00	6.270
Sardines, skinless, boneless, water pack	4	ea	84.00	182.00	.840
Scallops:					
Baked/broiled	4	ea	100.00	133.00	1.690
Battered, fried	10	ea	80.00	184.00	1.550
Breaded, fried	4.76	oz	135.00	290.00	3.240
Steamed/boiled	4.23	oz	120.00	128.00	1.620
Shark, baked/broiled	4.66	oz	132.00	236.00	2.160
Shark, batter fried	2	oz	56.70	129.00	1.130
Shrimp:					
Baked/broiled, med size	2	ea	10.00	15.50	.392
Batter fried	4.55	oz	129.00	312.00	5.130
Cake/patty	1	ea	120.00	248.00	2.700
Canned, drained	4.51	oz	128.00	154.00	3.200
Canned, not drained	3.5	oz	100.00	102.00	2.500
Prawn/large, breaded, frd	5	ea	85.00	206.00	3.380
Prawn/large, steamed/bld	10	ea	60.00	59.40	1.020
Smelt, floured/breaded, fried	2	ea	58.00	145.00	.872
Snail, steamed	2	ea	10.00	18.00	1.000
Sole/flounder:					
Batter fried	4	pce	64.00	121.00	1.040
Floured/breaded, fried	1	ea	81.00	176.00	2.220
Steamed/poached	4.66	oz	132.00	150.00	3.120
Squid:					
Baked/broiled	4.94	oz	140.00	193.00	2.700
Canned	6.6	oz	187.00	198.00	2.580

	Svg		Wt (g)	Cal	Vit E Alpha-Toc Eq
Meats: Fish & Shellfish, continued					
Fried in flour	5.29	oz	150.00	263.00	2.930
Pickled	2	oz	56.70	51.90	.654
Surimi (processed pollack)	2	oz	56.70	56.10	1.070
Trout, rainbow, farmed, cooked, dry heat	1	ea	71.00	120.00	1.950
Tuna:					
Fresh, floured/breaded, frd	4.66	oz	132.00	309.00	1.870
Fresh, smoked	4	pce	64.00	140.00	.960
Light, cnd, oil pack, drnd	1	ea	161.00	319.00	1.930
White, cnd, oil pack, drnd	1	ea	178.00	331.00	2.140

MEATS: POULTRY

	Svg		Wt (g)	Cal	Vit E Alpha-Toc Eq
Chicken:					
Back, w/skin, roasted	1	ea	53.00	159.00	.583
Gizzard, simmered	1	ea	22.00	33.70	.260
Liver, simmered	1	ea	20.00	31.40	.286
Neck, w/skin, flour fried	1	ea	36.00	120.00	.450
Wing:					
Flour fried	1	ea	32.00	103.00	.384
w/skin, batter fried	1	ea	49.00	159.00	.539
Goose, roasted:					
Skinless	4.97	oz	141.00	335.00	1.410
w/skin	4.97	oz	141.00	429.00	2.440
Turkey:					
Breast, w/skin, roasted	.5	ea	864.00	1632.00	18.000
Gizzard, simmered	1	ea	67.00	109.00	.844
Liver, simmered	1	ea	75.00	127.00	2.170

	Svg		Wt (g)	Cal	Vit E Alpha-Toc Eq

MIXED DISHES & FAST FOODS

	Svg		Wt (g)	Cal	Vit E Alpha-Toc Eq
Beef dishes:					
Curry	1	c	236.00	437.00	6.130
w/cream or white sauce	1	c	256.00	384.00	2.620
w/rice, w/tomato-based sce	1	c	244.00	338.00	3.180
Biscuits, fast food:					
w/egg+cheese+bacon	1	ea	144.00	477.00	1.440
w/egg+sausage	1	ea	180.00	581.00	2.160
w/sausage	1	ea	124.00	485.00	3.080
Chicken dishes:					
Almond chicken	1	c	242.00	275.00	2.640
Breast, w/cream sauce	1	ea	129.00	218.00	1.390
Curry	1	c	236.00	293.00	3.250
Kung pao	1	c	162.00	409.00	3.650
Parmigiana	1	pce	182.00	317.00	1.840
Patty, breaded, cooked	1	ea	75.00	213.00	1.460
Thigh, w/cream sauce	1	ea	78.00	132.00	.838
w/cream sauce	1	c	241.00	407.00	2.590
w/noodles in tomato sauce	1	c	224.00	286.00	2.380
w/rice, w/tomato-based sce	1	c	244.00	246.00	3.260
Chow mein/chop suey, shrimp:					
no noodles	1	c	220.00	172.00	2.800
w/noodles	1	c	220.00	277.00	2.540
Egg foo yung:					
Beef	1	ea	86.00	129.00	1.790
Chicken	1	ea	86.00	130.00	1.870
Pork	1	ea	86.00	134.00	1.870
Shrimp	1	ea	86.00	153.00	2.160
Egg omelet:					
1 lg egg+milk+butter	1	ea	59.00	89.70	.590
w/cheese+ham	1	ea	78.00	142.00	1.690
w/chicken	1	ea	95.00	149.00	2.080

	Svg		Wt (g)	Cal	Vit E Alpha-Toc Eq
Mixed Dishes & Fast Foods, continued					
w/dark grn vegetable	1	ea	84.00	94.70	1.690
w/fish	1	ea	88.00	132.00	2.120
w/mushroom	1	ea	69.00	91.20	1.530
w/onion, pepper, tomato, & mushroom	1	ea	145.00	125.00	1.880
w/sausage	1	ea	95.00	172.00	1.820
Egg roll, meatless	1	ea	64.00	102.00	.809
Egg roll, w/chicken	1	ea	64.00	105.00	.701
English muffin, fast food:					
w/egg+chse+Canadian bacon	1	ea	146.00	383.00	2.340
w/egg+cheese+sausage	1	ea	165.00	487.00	2.150
Grape leaves, stuffed:					
w/beef+rice	1	ea	21.00	52.90	.404
w/lamb+rice	1	ea	21.00	53.00	.450
Ham croquette	1	ea	62.00	152.00	.959
Ham/pork, w/tom-based sce	1	c	249.00	322.00	2.700
Liver, chopped (liver/egg/onion)	1	c	208.00	460.00	2.760
Liver dumpling	1	c	250.00	770.00	6.190
Liver pâté, goose, canned	1	T	13.00	60.10	.390
Manicotti, w/meat sauce	1	ea	233.00	304.00	1.510
Meat loaf, beef+1/3 pork	1	pce	87.00	221.00	.334
Oyster fritter	1	ea	40.00	125.00	.822
Pizza, cheese, 15", 1/8	1	pce	100.00	223.00	.685
Pot pie:					
Beef, recipe, baked	1	pce	210.00	517.00	3.780
Chicken, 1/3 recipe	1	pce	232.00	545.00	3.250
Chicken, f/frozen	1	ea	230.00	504.00	2.530
Ravioli, meat w/meat sauce	1	c	250.00	388.00	3.050
Ravioli, meat w/tomato sauce	2	ea	70.00	109.00	.853
Salads:					
Bean, yellow/green	1	c	150.00	140.00	1.960
Carrot raisin	1	c	175.00	404.00	9.820

	Svg		Wt (g)	Cal	Vit E Alpha-Toc Eq
Mixed Dishes & Fast Foods, continued					
Chicken, w/celery	.5	c	78.00	268.00	7.520
Coleslaw	1	c	120.00	178.00	4.800
Crab	1	c	208.00	284.00	2.860
Egg	1	c	183.00	586.00	8.870
Macaroni, no cheese	1	c	177.00	455.00	12.700
Potato	1	c	193.00	267.00	2.270
Salmon	1	c	208.00	407.00	5.210
Seafood	1	c	208.00	331.00	4.580
Spinach, no dressing	1	c	74.00	89.00	1.010
Waldorf	1	c	137.00	397.00	10.500
Salmon croquette	1	ea	63.00	137.00	1.110
Salmon loaf	1	ea	105.00	210.00	2.010
Sandwiches, on part wheat bread, unless otherwise indicated:					
Corned beef & Swiss, on rye	1	ea	147.00	457.00	3.940
Fish, w/cheese+tartar sauce	1	ea	183.00	523.00	3.480
Fish, w/tartar sauce	1	ea	158.00	431.00	3.000
Grilled cheese	1	ea	118.00	392.00	1.570
Ham	1	ea	123.00	259.00	2.580
Ham, on rye	1	ea	117.00	243.00	2.230
Ham & cheese	1	ea	152.00	387.00	3.340
Ham & swiss, on rye	1	ea	145.00	368.00	2.890
Patty melt, ground beef on rye	1	ea	177.00	600.00	4.620
Peanut butter & jam	1	ea	101.00	344.00	2.470
Roast beef	1	ea	123.00	314.00	3.410
Submarine ham & chse on roll	1	ea	219.00	532.00	2.410
Tuna salad	1	ea	117.00	329.00	4.470
Turkey	1	ea	123.00	269.00	3.540
Turkey ham	1	ea	122.00	255.00	2.790
Turkey ham, on rye	1	ea	116.00	239.00	2.450
Turkey ham & cheese	1	ea	152.00	385.00	3.530

	Svg		Wt (g)	Cal	Vit E Alpha-Toc Eq

Mixed Dishes & Fast Foods, continued
Shrimp dishes:

	Svg		Wt (g)	Cal	Vit E Alpha-Toc Eq
Cocktail	1	c	230.00	196.00	4.640
Creole, w/rice (jambalaya)	1	c	243.00	306.00	4.230
Curry	1	c	236.00	314.00	4.070
Salad	1	c	182.00	282.00	5.120
Sweet & sour	1	c	176.00	479.00	4.130
Teriyaki	1	c	201.00	250.00	4.890
w/noodles, w/cheese sce	1	c	224.00	350.00	4.770
Soufflé, cheese	1	c	112.00	195.00	1.270
Soufflé, seafood	1	c	159.00	258.00	2.990
Spaghetti, w/white clam sce	1	c	248.00	457.00	2.910
Stews: see Soups, Sauces & Gravies					
Taco, small	1	ea	171.00	369.00	1.880
Tortellini, spinach-filled, no sce	1	c	122.00	232.00	1.330
Tuna dishes:					
Loaf	1	ea	105.00	249.00	1.900
Noodle casserole	1	c	202.00	238.00	1.190
Noodle casserole, w/crm sce	1	c	224.00	432.00	2.650
w/cream or white sauce	1	c	237.00	411.00	3.220
Turkey patty, breaded, fried	1	ea	64.00	181.00	1.530
Veal parmigiana	7.25	oz	205.00	431.00	1.400
Veal scallopini	1	pce	96.00	257.00	2.200
Wonton, fried, meat filled	3	pce	57.00	183.00	1.720

NUTS & SEEDS

	Svg		Wt (g)	Cal	Vit E Alpha-Toc Eq
Almond butter, plain	1	T	15.60	98.90	3.170
Almond paste, packed	.5	c	114.00	508.00	23.100
Almonds:					
Blanched, sliced	1	c	105.00	615.00	5.880
Dried:					
Chopped	1	c	130.00	766.00	31.200
Slices	1	c	94.00	554.00	22.600

	Svg		Wt (g)	Cal	Vit E Alpha-Toc Eq
Nuts & Seeds, continued					
Slivered, packed	1	c	135.00	795.00	32.400
Whole	1	c	142.00	836.00	34.100
Dry roasted	1	c	138.00	810.00	7.660
Salted	1	c	138.00	810.00	33.100
Oil roasted, blanched	1	c	142.00	871.00	36.900
Roasted	1	c	157.00	970.00	41.600
Whole, toasted	1	oz	28.40	167.00	6.620
Brazil nut, dried	1	c	140.00	918.00	10.600
Cashew, oil roasted	1	c	130.00	749.00	2.030
Cashew butter	1	T	16.00	93.90	.250
Chestnut, dried, peeled	1	oz	28.40	105.00	.567
Chestnut, European, roasted	17	ea	143.00	350.00	1.720
Coconut, dried:					
Shredded, sweetened	1	c	93.00	466.00	.744
Toasted	1	oz	28.40	168.00	.284
Unsweetened	1	c	78.00	515.00	1.090
Coconut cream, raw	1	c	240.00	792.00	2.640
Filberts/hazelnuts:					
Dried:					
Blanched	2	oz	56.70	381.00	14.600
Chopped	1	c	115.00	727.00	27.500
Whole	1	c	135.00	853.00	32.300
Dry roasted	2	oz	56.70	375.00	14.200
Oil roasted	2	oz	56.70	374.00	14.200
Gingko nut, canned	1	c	155.00	172.00	5.430
Ginkgo nut, dried	1	oz	28.40	98.70	1.220
Hickory nut, dried	1	oz	28.40	186.00	1.480
Macadamias, oil roasted:	11	ea	28.40	204.00	.992
Chopped	1	c	110.00	790.00	3.850
Salted	1	c	134.00	962.00	4.690
Mixed nuts:					
Dry roasted, w/peanuts	1	c	137.00	814.00	8.220

	Svg		Wt (g)	Cal	Vit E Alpha-Toc Eq
Oil roasted, w/o peanuts	1	c	144.00	886.00	8.640
Oil roasted, w/peanuts	1	c	142.00	876.00	8.520
Peanut butter	2	T	32.00	189.00	2.400
Natural	2	T	32.00	187.00	2.590
Peanuts:					
Boiled, edible part	1	c	62.90	200.00	2.330
Dry roasted	1	c	146.00	854.00	10.800
Oil roasted	1	c	144.00	837.00	10.700
Spanish, oil roasted	1	c	147.00	851.00	10.900
Spanish, raw	1	c	146.00	832.00	10.800
Valencia, oil roasted	1	c	144.00	848.00	11.400
Virginia, dry	1	c	145.00	822.00	12.100
Virginia, oil roasted	1	c	143.00	827.00	10.400
Pecans:					
Dried, chopped	1	c	119.00	794.00	3.690
Dried, halves	1	c	108.00	720.00	3.350
Dry roasted	1	c	114.00	748.00	3.410
Oil roasted	1	c	110.00	754.00	3.630
Pine nut, dried (pignolia)	1	oz	28.40	146.00	2.720
Pine nut, dried (piñon/pinyon)	1	oz	28.40	161.00	.992
Pistachio, dry roasted	1	c	128.00	776.00	6.670
Pumpkin seed kernel, dry rstd	1	c	138.00	747.00	1.380
Pumpkin seed kernel, roasted	1	c	227.00	1184.00	2.270
Sesame butter/tahini, f/roasted, toasted kernels	1	T	15.00	89.30	.341
Sesame seed, kernel, toasted	1	oz	28.00	159.00	.613
Sesame seed, whl, rstd, tstd	1	T	8.88	50.10	.202
Soy nuts/soybeans, rstd, kernel	.5	c	86.00	390.00	1.680
f/dry	.5	c	86.00	387.00	3.960
Sunflower seed butter	1	T	16.00	92.60	7.680
Sunflower seeds, kernels:					
Dry	1	c	144.00	820.00	72.400
Dry roasted	1	c	128.00	745.00	64.400

	Svg		Wt (g)	Cal	Vit E Alpha-Toc Eq
Nuts & Seeds, continued					
Oil roasted	1	c	135.00	830.00	67.900
Toasted	1	c	134.00	830.00	76.800
Walnuts, dried:					
Black, chopped	1	c	125.00	759.00	3.280
English, chopped	1	c	120.00	770.00	3.140
English, halves	1	c	100.00	642.00	2.620

SOUPS, SAUCES & GRAVIES

	Svg		Wt (g)	Cal	Vit E Alpha-Toc Eq
Sauces: see also Miscellaneous					
Cheese	.5	c	101.00	216.00	1.230
Curry	.5	c	115.00	74.40	.815
Hollandaise	1	c	160.00	684.00	2.470
Marinara, canned	1	c	250.00	170.00	4.000
Mornay	.5	c	172.00	429.00	2.260
Spaghetti:					
Canned	1	c	249.00	271.00	4.980
Meat, canned	1	c	250.00	300.00	5.910
w/beef, recipe	1	c	248.00	289.00	4.280
w/meatballs, canned	1	c	250.00	255.00	4.000
w/mushrooms, canned	.75	c	185.00	162.00	2.040
w/mushrooms, recipe	.75	c	185.00	108.00	1.640
White, medium, recipe	1	c	250.00	355.00	3.390
Soups:					
Bouillabaisse	1	c	227.00	242.00	2.290
Stew, Brunswick	1	c	250.00	174.00	.392
Stew, seafood, w/potato & veg	1	c	252.00	169.00	2.530
Tomato, w/milk	1	c	248.00	161.00	2.600
Tomato, w/water	1	c	244.00	85.40	2.490

	Svg		Wt (g)	Cal	Vit E Alpha-Toc Eq

VEGETABLES & LEGUMES

	Svg		Wt (g)	Cal	Vit E Alpha-Toc Eq
Artichoke heart, marinated	1	c	130.00	128.00	1.430
Asparagus, pieces:					
Boiled	.5	c	90.00	21.60	.900
Canned, drained	.5	c	121.00	23.00	1.210
Frozen, boiled	1	c	180.00	50.40	2.430
Steamed/stir-fried, no oil	1	c	180.00	41.40	3.600
Beet greens, boiled	1	c	144.00	38.90	2.020
Broccoli pieces, boiled	1	c	156.00	43.70	1.720
Cabbage:					
Common:					
Boiled, shredded	1	c	150.00	33.00	2.490
Shredded	1	c	70.00	17.50	1.170
Steamed/stir-fried, no oil	1	c	150.00	37.50	2.480
Pak choi, boiled	.5	c	85.00	10.20	1.450
Red	1	c	70.00	18.90	1.170
Savoy	1	c	70.00	18.90	1.170
Savoy, boiled, drained	1	c	145.00	34.80	2.410
Carrot, cooked, glazed	1	c	161.00	234.00	2.310
Cauliflower, batter-dipped, frd	5	pce	130.00	250.00	3.430
Dandelion greens	1	c	55.00	24.80	1.380
Dandelion greens, boiled, drnd	1	c	105.00	34.70	2.100
Jicama/yambean	1	c	120.00	45.60	5.480
Jicama/yambean, ckd slice	1	c	100.00	38.00	4.500
Kale, chopped	1	c	67.00	33.50	.670
Mushroom, batter-dipped, fried	5	ea	70.00	148.00	.919
Mustard green	1	c	56.00	14.60	1.130
Mustard green, boiled, drained	1	c	140.00	21.00	2.810
Okra, batter-dipped, fried	1	c	92.00	175.00	3.090
Pepper, jalapeño, cnd, not drnd	.5	c	68.00	16.30	1.360
Pumpkin, canned	.5	c	123.00	41.80	1.290
Sauerkraut, canned, not drnd	1	c	236.00	44.80	3.940

	Svg		Wt (g)	Cal	Vit E Alpha-Toc Eq
Vegetables & Legumes, *continued*					
Seaweed, wakame	1	c	80.00	36.00	1.760
Soybean greens	.5	c	128.00	188.00	1.920
Soybean greens, boiled, drnd	.5	c	90.00	127.00	1.260
Soybeans, dry, boiled	1	c	172.00	298.00	3.340
Soy flour, full fat, raw	1	c	85.00	371.00	1.660
Soy Products: see also Dairy, Nuts & Seeds, Vegetarian Foods					
Spinach:					
Boiled, drained	1	c	180.00	41.40	2.340
Boiled, f/frozen, drained	1	c	190.00	53.20	2.000
Canned, drained	1	c	214.00	49.20	5.350
Raw	1	c	56.00	12.30	.974
Steamed	.5	c	95.00	20.90	1.800
Stir-fried	1	c	180.00	39.60	3.400
Sweet potatoes:					
Baked, peel eaten	1	ea	77.00	94.90	2.740
Candied	1	c	196.00	269.00	7.450
Canned, w/syrup, drained	1	c	196.00	212.00	11.800
Swiss chard, chopped	1	c	36.00	6.84	.626
Taro, Tahitian, cooked slice	1	c	137.00	60.30	4.110
Taro shoot, cooked slice	1	c	140.00	19.60	1.400
Tomatillo, chopped	.5	c	66.00	21.10	.660
Tomatoes:					
Green, fried	1	ea	144.00	238.00	1.930
Red, fried	1	ea	101.00	164.00	1.350
Sun-dried	1	c	54.00	139.00	1.620
Tomato paste, canned	1	c	262.00	220.00	5.660
Tomato sauce w/onion, green pepper, & celery, canned	1	c	245.00	101.00	2.450
Turnip green, boiled	1	c	144.00	28.80	2.460
Turnip green, chopped	1	c	55.00	14.90	1.230
Yam, white, boiled/baked	1	c	136.00	158.00	6.200

	Svg		Wt (g)	Cal	Vit E Alpha-Toc Eq

VEGETARIAN FOODS

	Svg		Wt (g)	Cal	Vit E Alpha-Toc Eq
Bacon, simulated meat	3	ea	24.00	74.40	1.660
Bacon bits, meatless	4	ea	57.00	253.00	3.930
Breakfast links	1	ea	25.00	64.00	.525
Breakfast patties	1	ea	38.00	97.30	.798
Chicken, meatless	2	ea	60.00	132.00	1.610
Chicken, meatless, brd, fried	1	pce	57.00	96.90	1.110
Chili made w/meat substitute	.66	c	141.00	186.00	1.640
Fillet	1	ea	47.00	136.00	1.620
Frankfurter, meatless	1	ea	51.00	102.00	.979
Luncheon slice, meatless	1	pce	67.00	188.00	2.010
Meatball, meatless	7	ea	70.00	140.00	1.210
Meat loaf/patties	1	oz	28.00	56.00	.484
Scallops, meatless, brd, fried	.5	c	85.00	257.00	3.500
Soyburger	1	ea	71.00	142.00	1.230
Soyburger w/cheese	1	ea	135.00	316.00	1.430

MISCELLANEOUS

	Svg		Wt (g)	Cal	Vit E Alpha-Toc Eq
Banana, choc-covered, w/nuts	1	ea	145.00	336.00	1.920
Bean dip, w/refried beans	1	c	262.00	365.00	3.010
Candy:					
Almond, chocolate-coated	1	c	165.00	937.00	20.800
Hershey's Kisses	6	pce	28.40	145.00	.352
M&M's, peanut	10	pce	20.00	99.00	.620
M&M's, plain	10	pce	7.00	33.30	.070
Peanut, milk-choc-covered	1	c	170.00	882.00	6.460
Peanut, yogurt-covered	1	c	170.00	774.00	8.160
Peanut brittle, recipe	1	c	147.00	666.00	2.410
Toffee, choc-coated, w/nuts	1	pce	11.00	48.40	.171
Toffee, recipe	1	pce	12.00	65.00	.240

	Svg		Wt (g)	Cal	Vit E Alpha-Toc Eq
Miscellaneous, continued					
Candy bars:					
Alpine White, w/almonds	1	ea	35.00	193.00	1.330
Baby Ruth	1	ea	60.00	281.00	1.920
Bar None	1	ea	42.00	219.00	.512
Butterfinger	1	ea	61.00	286.00	.793
Milk chocolate	1	ea	44.00	226.00	.546
Mr. Goodbar	1	ea	49.00	252.00	1.470
Skor English toffee	1	ea	39.00	206.00	.534
Snickers	1	ea	58.70	267.00	1.230
Sweet chocolate	1	ea	41.00	207.00	.488
Symphony	1	ea	42.00	219.00	.521
Whatchamacallit	1	ea	48.00	241.00	1.920
Chocolate, sweet dark	1	oz	28.40	135.00	.337
Chocolate chips, milk choc	1	c	170.00	872.00	2.110
Chocolate chips, semisweet	1	c	170.00	811.00	2.020
Condiments:					
Guacamole, w/tomatoes	1	c	233.00	278.00	2.380
Hummus/hummous, raw	1	c	246.00	421.00	7.350
Olive, green, no pits	10	ea	39.00	45.20	1.170
Olive, large, canned	10	ea	45.00	51.70	1.040
Oyster sauce, bottled	1	c	256.00	289.00	3.410
Pesto sauce	1	c	232.00	1242.00	11.600
Picante sauce, Tostitos	6	T	85.00	40.00	1.930
Steak sce, tom-based (A-1)	1	c	250.00	153.00	4.340
Tartar sauce	1	T	14.00	74.30	2.240
Tartar sauce, low calorie	1	T	14.00	30.80	.831
Rice Krispies bar	1	ea	28.00	109.00	.425
Yogurt chips	1	oz	28.00	146.00	.691

NOTES

INTRODUCTION: VITAMIN E, YOUR GREAT PROTECTOR

1. Lawrence Kushi et al., "Dietary Antioxidant Vitamins and Death from Coronary Heart Disease in Postmenopausal Women," *New England Journal of Medicine* 334 (1996): 1156–62.
2. William J. Blot, "Vitamin/Mineral Supplementation and Cancer Risk: Findings from a Randomized Trial in China," presented at the American Association for Cancer Research 85th Annual Meeting, San Francisco, California, April 11, 1994.
3. P. Knekt et al., "Serum Antioxidant Vitamins and Risk of Cataract," *British Medical Journal* 305 (1992): 1392–94; Johanna Seddon et al., *American Journal of Public Health* 84, no. 5 (May 1994): 788–92.
4. Jan Breslow, president of the American Heart Association, "Top Ten Research Advances in Heart Disease, 1996," press release, December 18, 1996, Dallas, Texas; Rebecca Voelker, "Recommendations for Antioxidants: How Much Evidence Is Enough?" *Journal of the American Medical Association* 271, no. 15 (April 20, 1994): 1148–50.

1: THE DISCOVERY

1. H. Evans and K. S. Bishop, "On the Existence of Hitherto Unrecognized Dietary Factor Essential for Reproduction," *Science* 56 (1922): 650–51.

2. "Paul Gyorgy—An Appreciation, April 7, 1893–March 1, 1976," *Nutrition Review* 34, no. 5 (May 1976): 159–60.

3. J. Sanquansermsri, P. Gyorgy, and F. Zilliken, "Polyamines in Human and Cow's Milk," *American Journal of Clinical Nutrition* 27, no. 8 (August 1996): 859–65.

4. M. K. Horwitt, "Therapuetic Uses of Vitamin E in Medicine," *Nutrition Reviews* 38 (1980): 105–13.

5. K. Pietrzik, "Concept of Borderline Vitamin Deficiencies," *International Journal of Vitamin and Nutrition Research* Supplement 27 (1985): 61–73.

6. H. J. Powers, Bates et al., "Running Performance in Gambian Children: Effects of Water-Soluble Vitamins or Iron," *European Journal of Clinical Nutrition* 42, no. 11 (November 1988): 895–902; C. J. Dillard et al., "Effects of Exercise, Vitamin and Ozone on Pulmonary Function and Lipid Peroxidation," *Journal of Applied Physiology* 45 (1978): 927–32; E. J. Vanderbeek et al., "Impact of Marginal Vitamin Intake on Physiological Performance in Healthy Young Men," *Proceedings of the Nutrition Society* 44 (1985): 27A.

7. R. Buzina, "Marginal Malnutrition and Its Functional Consequences in Industrialized Societies," *Progress in Clinical Biological Research* 77 (1981): 285–303.

8. David Stipp, "Studies Showing Benefits of Antioxidants Prove Potent Tonic for Sales of Vitamin E," *Wall Street Journal,* April 13, 1993, B1.

2: THE SHADY LADY FIGHTS YOUR FREE RADICALS

1. Balz Frei, Laura England, and Bruce Ames, "Ascorbate Is an Outstanding Antioxidant in Human Blood Plasma," *Proceedings of the National Academy of Sciences* 86 (August 1989): 6377–81.

3: VITAMIN E AND YOUR BLOOD

1. L. Corash et al., "Reduced Chronic Hemolysis During High-Dose Vitamin E Administration in Mediterranean-Type Glucose-6-Phosphate Dehydrogenase Deficient Kurdish and Iraqi Males," *American Journal of Clinical Nutrition* 34 (1981): 626.

2. B. S. Baglia et al., "Chemoluminescence Response of Polymorphonuclear Leukocytes from Vitamin E Deficient Sickle-Cell Patients," *Nutrition Reports International* 39 (1989): 761–71.

3. C. L. Natta, L. J. Machlin, and M. Brin, "A Decrease in Irreversibly Sickled Erthyrocytes in Sickle-Cell Anemia Patients Given Vitamin E," *American Journal of Clinical Nutrition,* 33 (1980): 968–71.

4. G. M. Rubanyi, "Vascular Effects of Oxygen-Derived Free Radicals," *Free Radical Biological Medicine* 4 (1988): 107–20.

5. L. Packer, E. H. Witt, and H. J. Tritschler, "Alpha-Lipoic Acid as a Biological Antioxidant," *Free Radical Biological Medicine* 19, no. 2 (August 1995): 227–50.

6. J. T. Salonen et al., "Increased Oxidation Resistance of Atherogenic Plasma Lipoproteins at High Vitamin E Levels in Non-Vitamin E Supplemented Men," Atherosclerosis 124, no. 1 (July 1996): 83–94.

7. Maury Breecher, personal communication with author, January 24, 1997.

8. P. Dowd, and Z. B. Zhang, "On the Mechanism of the Anticlotting Action of Vitamin E Quinone," *Proceedings of the National Academy of Sciences* 92, no. 18 (August 29, 1995): 8171–75.

9. S. Renaud et al., "Influence of Vitamin E Administration on Platelet Functions in Hormonal Contraceptive Users," *Contraception* 36 (1987): 347–58; M. J. Stampfer et al., "Vitamin E Supplementation Effect on Human Platelet Function, Arachidonic Acid Metabolism and Plasma Prostacyclin Levels," *American Journal of Clinical Nutrition* 47 (1995): 700–706.

10. N. C. Cavarocchi et al., Superoxide Generation During Cardiopulmonary Bypass: Is There a Role for Vitamin E? *Journal of Surgical Research* 40 (1986): 519–27.

4: VITAMIN E AND YOUR HEART

1. Breslow, "Top Ten Research Advances."
2. N. G. Stephens et al., "Randomized Controlled Trial of Vitamin E in Patients with Coronary Disease: Cambridge Heart Antioxidant Study (CHAOS), (1996): 781 *Lancet* 347; R. A. Riemer "Coronary Heart Disease and Vitamin E" (editorial), Ibid., 776.
3. Stephens, "Randomized Controlled Trial of Vitamin E."
4. K. F. Gey, "Prospects for the Prevention of Free Radical Disease, Regarding Cancer and Cardiovascular Disease," *British Medical Bulletin* 49 (1993): 679–99.
5. Kushi et al., "Dietary Antioxidant Vitamins."
6. E. B. Rimm et al., "Vitamin E Consumption and the Risk of Coronary Disease in Men," *New England Journal of Medicine* 328 (1993): 1444–49.
7. Mohsen Meydani, "Vitamin E," *Lancet* 345 (January 21, 1995): 170–76; J. T. Salonen et al., "Serum Fatty Acids Apolipoproteins, Selenium, and Vitamin Antioxidants and Risk of Death from Coronary Artery Disease," *American Journal of Cardiology* 56 (1985): 226–31.
8. M. C. Bellizzi et al., "Vitamin E and Coronary Heart Disease: the European Paradox," *European Journal of Clinical Nutrition* 48, no. 11 (November 1994): 822–31.
9. Paul Dudley White, "Atherosclerosis," *Clinician,* a medical journal published by Searle, in 1972.
10. Ishwarlal Jialal, "Influence of Antioxidant Vitamins on LDL Oxidation," paper presented at New York Academy of Sciences meeting, New York, New York, December 1996.
11. American Heart Association Journal News Briefs, Dallas, Texas, September 15, 1996.

12. Ishwarlal Jialal et al., *Journal of Lipid Research* 33 (1992): 899–906.

13. Ishwarlal Jialal, "Scientist Notes Novel Action of Vitamin E in Preventing Atherosclerotic Plaque," Southwestern Medical Center research, August 7, 1996, Dallas, Texas.

14. S. Devaraj, D. Li, and I. Jialal, *Journal of Clinical Investigation* 98 (1996): 756–63.

15. Iswarlal Jialal, personal communication with author, March 24, 1997.

16. T. M. Yau et al., "Vitamin E for Coronary Bypass Operations: A Prospective Double-Blind, Randomized Trial," *Journal of Thoracic and Cardiovascular Surgery* 108, no. 2 (August 1994): 302–10.

17. D. R. Jancro, "Therapeutic Potential of Vitamin E Against Myocardial Ischemic-Reperfusion Injury," *Free Radical Biology and Medicine* 10 (1991): 315–24; Cavarocchi et al., "Superoxide Generation During Cardiopulmonary Bypass."

18. Kunihisa Miwa et al., "Vitamin E Deficiency in Variant Angina," *Circulation* 94 (1996): 14–18.

19. R. A. Riemersma et al., "Risk of Angina Pectoris and Plasma Concentrations of Vitamin A, C, and E and Carotene," *Lancet* 337 (1991): 8732.

20. Janne Rapola et al., "Effect of Vitamin E and Beta-Carotene on the Incidence of Angina Pectoris," *Journal of the American Medical Association* 275, no. 9 (March 6, 1996): 693–98.

21. K. Haeger, "Long-Term Study of Alpha Tocopherol in Intermittent Claudication," *Annals of New York Academy of Sciences* 393 (1982): 369–75.

22. L. E. Chambless, E. Shahar, and J. Toole, "Association of Transient Ischemic Attack/Stroke Symptoms Assessed by Standardized Questionnaire and Algorithm with Cerebrovascular Risk Factors and Carotid Artery Wall Thickness: The ARIC Study, 1987–1989," *American Journal of Epidemiology* 144, no. 9 (November 1, 1996): 857–66; *Newswire,* Winston-Salem, North Carolina, October 30, 1996.

23. Stephen Kritchevsky et al., "Dietary Antioxidants and Carotid

Artery Wall Thickness: The ARIC Study," *Circulation* 92 (1995): 2142–50.

24. American Diabetes Association, "Diabetes Facts," January 1997, New York, New York.

25. C. Fuller et al., *American Journal of Clinical Nutrition,* May 1996.

26. "Vitamin E Appears to Reduce Risk of Heart Disease in Diabetics," *Southwestern News,* Dallas, Texas, April 28, 1996.

27. Jialal, personal communication with author.

28. Antonio Ceriello et al., "Vitamin E Reduction of Protein Glycosylation in Diabetes," *Diabetes Care* 14, no. 1 (January 1991).

29. Sven-Erik Bursell on "Diabetic Retinopathy and Vitamin E," paper presented at a scientific symposium sponsored by the American Diabetes Association, November 29, 1996.

30. G. Paolisso et al., *Diabetes Care* 16 (1993): 1433–37.

31. Jukka Salonen et al., "Increased Risk of Non-Insulin-Dependent Diabetes Mellitus at Low Plasma Vitamin E Concentrations: A Four-Year Follow-up Study in Men," *British Medical Journal* 311 (October 28, 1995): 1124–27.

32. G. Plotnick, M. Corretti, and R. Vogel, "Vitamin C and Vitamin E May Counter Effects of Oxygen-Free Radicals on Arteries," paper presented to the American Heart Association's 69th Scientific Session, New Orleans, November 12, 1996.

33. Farzin Fath-Ordoubadi, letter to the editor, *Lancet* 347 (June 15, 1996): 1689.

34. Nigel G. Stephens, letter to the editor on behalf of the CHAOS investigators, *Lancet* 347 (June 15, 1996): 1690.

35. Kofo Ogunyankin, letter to the editor, *Lancet* 347 (June 15, 1996): 1689.

36. Mary Burnette, "Vitamin E: Star Nutrient of 1996" (news release), Council for Responsible Nutrition, Washington, D.C., December 19, 1996.

37. M. J. Stampfer and E. B. Rimm, "Epidemiologic Evidence for Vitamin E in Prevention of Cardiovascular Disease," *American Jour-*

nal of Clinical Nutrition 62, no. 6 Suppl. (December 1995): 1365–69S.

38. "Research Focuses on Role of Vitamins in Heart Disease," *Lahey Clinic Health Letter,* September 1993, 1.
39. Burnette, "Vitamin E: Star Nutrient."
40. American Heart Association 1997 Heart and Stroke Statistical Update, Dallas, Texas.

5: VITAMIN E AND CANCER

1. "Highlights of National Cancer Institute's Carcinogenesis Studies," National Institutes of Health, June 25, 1993.
2. Robert J. Scheuplein, "Perspectives on Toxicological Risk—an Example: Foodborne Carcinogenic Risk," *Critical Reviews of Food Science and Nutrition* 32, no. 2 (1992): 105–21.
3. Suzanne Gaby et al., *Vitamin Intake and Health: A Scientific Review* (New York: Marcel Dekker, 1991), 73.
4. S. L. Haber and R. W. Wissler, "Effect of Vitamin E on the Carcinogenicity of Methylcholanthrene," *Proceedings of the Society for Experimental Biological Medicine* 111 (1962): 744.
5. S. S. Epstein et al., "The Null Effect of Antioxidants on the Carcinogenicity of 3,4,9-10-dibenzypyrene to Mice," *Life Sciences* 6 (1967): 225.
6. R. E. Olson, "The Function and Metabolism of Vitamin K: Review Article," *Annual Review of Nutrition* 4 (1987): 281–337.
7. Y. Kishino, and S. Moriguchi, "Nutritional Factors and Cellular Immune Responses," *Nutritional Health* 8, nos. 2–3 (1992): 133–41.
8. *Lung Disease Data 1996* (New York: American Lung Association): 16.
9. H. T. Madabushi, C. L. De Mulder, and A. L. Tappel, "Vitamin E Protects Chick Tissues Against In Vivo Oxidation of Heme Protein," *Lipids* 31, no. 1 (January 1996): 43–46; C. A. Knudsen, L. Tappel, and J. North, "Multiple Antioxidants Protect Against

Heme Protein and Lipid Oxidation in Kidney Tissue," *Free Radical Biologic Medicine,* no. 2 (1996): 165–73.

10. Jan Ehrman, "High Vitamin E Intake May Help Thwart Colon Cancer," *National Institutes of Health News & Features,* January/February 1994.

11. Ruth Winter, *A Consumer's Dictionary of Food Additives,* (New York: Crown, 1994): 281.

12. Ibid.

13. Ibid.

14. L. Packer and M. G. Traber, "Vitamin E: Beyond Antioxidant Function," *American Journal of Clinical Nutrition* 62, Suppl. 6 (December 1995): 1501S–1509S.

15. O. E. Odeleye et al., "Vitamin E Protection Against Nitrosamine-Induced Esophageal Tumor Incidence in Mice Immunocompromised by Retroviral Infection," *Carcinogenesis* 13, no. 10 (October 1992): 1811–16.

16. Ruth Winter, *Poisons in Your Food,* (New York: Crown, 1991): 90–91.

17. William Blot, "Diet and Cancer: The Role of Protective Factors," paper presented at the American Association for Cancer Research 85th Annual Meeting, San Francisco, April 11, 1994.

18. Paul Knekt et al., "Serum Vitamin E and Risk of Cancer among Finnish Men During a 10-Year Follow-up," *American Journal of Epidemiology* 127, no. 1, (1988): 28–41.

19. G. Gridley et al., "Vitamin Supplement Use and Reduced Risk of Oral and Pharyngeal Cancer," *American Journal of Epidemiology* 135, no. 10 (May 15, 1992): 1083–92.

20. J. K. McLaughlin et al., "Dietary Factors in Oral and Pharyngeal Cancer," *Journal of the National Cancer Institute* 80, no. 5 (October 5, 1988): 1237–43.

21. Packer and Traber, "Vitamin E."

22. Larry Clarke et al., "Selenium May Help Prevent Certain Types of Cancers," *Journal of the American Medical Association,* December 25, 1996.

6: VITAMIN E AND MUSCLE POWER

1. Ji, Li Li, "Oxidative Stress During Exercise: Implication of Antioxidant Nutrients," *Free Radical Biology & Medicine* 18, no. 6 (1995): 1079–86.

2. A. Hartman et al., "Vitamin E Prevents Exercise-Induced DNA Damage," *Mutation Research* 346, no. 4 (April 1995): 195–202.

3. J. G. Cannon et al., "Acute Phase Response in Exercise. II. Associations between Vitamin E, Cytokines, and Muscle Proteolysis," *American Journal of Physiology* 260, no. 6, pt. 2 (June 1991): R1235–40.

4. S. N. Meydani et al., "Protective Effect of Vitamin E on Exercise-Induced Oxidative Damage in Young and Older Adults," *American Journal of Physiology* 264 (Regulatory Integrative Comp. Physiology 33) (1993): R992–98.

5. Phyllis Clarkson, "Antioxidants and Physical Performance," *Critical Reviews in Food Science and Nutrition* 35 nos. 1 & 2 (1995): 131–41.

6. I. Simon-Schnass et al., "Effect of Vitamin E on Exercise Parameters in High Altitude Mountaineering," *Seutsch Z. Sportmedi* 38 (1987): 200–206.

7. Gaby et al., *Vitamin Intake and Health* 87–88.

8. L. A. Leschchinskii et al., "Experience in Using Helium-Neon Laser Irradiation Alone and in the Combined Therapy of Myocardial Infarct and Other Forms of IHD," *Ter Arkh* 67, no. 12 (1995): 13–17.

9. J. D. Riley and S. J. Antony, "Leg Cramps: Differential Diagnosis and Management," *American Family Physician* 53, no. 6 (1995): 1794–98.

10. Packer and Traber, "Vitamin E: Beyond Antioxidant Function."

11. H. F. Hintz, Review article, *Journal of Nutrition* 124, no. 12 (Suppl.) (December 1994): 2723S–29S; S. M. Somani and C. M. Arroyo, "Exercise Training Generates Ascorbate Free Radical in

Rat Heart," *Indiana Journal of Physiology and Pharmacology* 39, no. 4 (October 1995): 323–29.

12. Packer and Traber, "Vitamin E: Beyond Antioxidant Function."

13. W. J. Kraemer, S. J. Fleck, and W. J. Evans, "Strength and Power Training: Physiological Mechanisms of Adaptation," *Exercise Sports Science Review* 24 (1996): 363–97.

14. W. J. Evans, interview with author, March 17, 1997.

15. J. S. Dekkers et al., "The Role of Antioxidant Vitamins and Enzymes in the Prevention of Exercise-Induced Muscle Damage," *Sports Medicine* 21, no. 3 (March 1996): 213–38.

16. Somani and Arroyo, "Exercise Training Generates Ascorbate Free Radical."

17. P. M. Tidus et al., "Lack of Antioxidant Adaptation to Short-Term Aerobic Training in Human Muscle," *American Journal of Physiology* 271, no. 4, pt. 2 (October 1996): R832–36; L. Avellini et al., "Training-Induced Modification in Some Biochemical Defenses Against Free Radicals in Equine Erythrocytes," *Veterinary Research Communication* 19, no. 3 (1995): 179–84; P. C. Sharpe et al., "Total Radical Trapping Antioxidant Potential (TRAP) and Exercise," *Oxford Journal of Medicine* 89, no. 3 (March 1996): 223–28.

18. K. J. A. Davies et al., "Free Radicals and Tissue Damage Produced by Exercise," *Biochemistry and Biophysical Research Communication* 107 (1982): 1198–1205.

19. C. J. Dillard et al., "Effects of Exercise, Vitamin E and Ozone on Pulmonary Function and Lipid Peroxidation," *Journal of Applied Physiology* 45 (1978): 927–32.

20. R. A. Jacob and B. J. Burri, "Oxidative Damage and Defense," *American Journal of Clinical Nutrition* 63, no. 6 (June 1996): 985S–90S.

21. P. M. Tidus and Houston, "Vitamin E Status and Response to Exercise Training," *Sports Medicine* 20, no. 1 (July 1995): 12–23.

22. J. D. Riley and S. J. Antony, "Leg Cramps: Differential Diagnosis and Management," *American Family Physician* 52, no. 6 (November 1, 1995): 1794–98.

23. S. Ayres and R. Mihan, "Leg Cramps (Systremma) and 'Restless Legs' Syndrome. Response to Vitamin E (Tocopherol)," *California Medicine* 111, no. 2 (1996): 87–91.

24. R. F. Cathcart 3rd, "Leg Cramps and Vitamin E" (a letter), *Journal of the American Medical Association* 219, no. 2 (1972): 216–17.

7: VITAMIN E AND YOUR LUNGS

1. J. R. Britton et al., "Dietary Antioxidant Vitamin Intake and Lung Function in the General Population," *American Journal of Respiratory and Critical Care Medicine* 151 (1995): 1383–87.

2. R. J. Troisi, et al., "A Prospective Study of Diet and Adult-Onset Asthma," *American Journal of Respiratory and Critical Care Management* 151 (1995): 1401–8.

3. O. J. Carey et al., "The Effect of Lifestyle on Wheeze, Atopy, and Bronchial Hyperactivity in Asian and White Children," *American Journal of Respiratory and Critical Care Medicine* 153 (1996): 537–40.

4. M. Kamimura, "Anti-inflammatory Activity of Vitamin E," *Journal of Vitaminology* 18, no. 4 (1972): 204–9.

5. Lindsey Dow, "Does Dietary Intake of Vitamins C and E Influence Lung Function in Older People?" *The American Journal of Respiratory and Critical Care Medicine* (November 1995): 1401–4.

6. Packer and Traber, "Vitamin E: Beyond Antioxidant Function."

7. R. Shariff et al., "Vitamin E Supplementation in Smokers," *American Journal of Clinical Nutrition* 47 (1988): 758.

8: VITAMIN E AND YOUR SKIN

1. F. Nachbar and H. C. Korting, "The Role of Vitamin E in Normal and Damaged Skin," *Journal of Molecular Medicine* 73, no. 1 (January 1995): 7–17.

2. W. Pryor, *Free Radicals in Biology,* vol. 1 (New York: Academic Press, 1976): chapter 1.

3. I. Record et al., "The Influence of Topical and Synthetic Vitamin

E on Ultraviolet Light-Induced Skin Damage in Hairless Mice," *Nutrition and Cancer,* 16 (1991): 219–22; M. Roshupkin et al., "Inhibition of Ultraviolet Light-Induced Erythema by Antioxidants," *Archives of Dermatology Research* 266 (1979): 91–94; A. Potapenko et al., PUVA-Induced Erythema Changes in Mechano-Electrical Properties of Skin and Inhibition by Tocopherols," *Archives of Dermatology* 278, no. 1 (1984): 12–16. G. DeRios et al., "Systemic Protection by Antioxidants Against UVL-Induced Erythema," *Journal of Investigative Dermatology* 70 (1978): 123–25.

4. Elia Ben-Ari, "Research Briefings: Sun and Skin," National Institute of Arthritis and Musculoskeletal and Skin Diseases, Bethesda, Maryland, August 1993.

5. D. Darr et al., "Effectiveness of Antioxidants (Vitamin C and Vitamin E) Without Sunscreens as Topical Photoprotectants," *Acta Dermato-Venereologica,* 76, no. 4 (July 1996): 264–68.

6. H. L. Gensler et al., "Importance of the Form of Topical Vitamin E for Prevention of Photocarcinogenesis," *Nutrition and Cancer* 26, no. 2 (1996): 183–91.

7. T. Watabiki, *Vitamins* (Japan) 49 (1975): 121.

8. David Djerassi, Lawrence Machlin, and Carol Nocka, "Vitamin E Biochemical Function and Its Role in Cosmetics," *Drug and Cosmetic Industry,* March 1986, 6–9.

9. Ibid.

10. M. Erlich et al., "Inhibitory Effect of Vitamin E on Collagen Synthesis and Wound Repair," *Annals of Surgery* 175, no. 2 (February, 1972).

11. M. Kaminura and J. Matsuzawa, "Percutaneous Absorption of Alpha Tochopheryl Acetate," *Journal of Vitaminology* 14 (1963): 150–59.

12. Ibid.

13. New York Academy of Science Conference: "Vitamin E Biochemistry and Health Implications," October 31–November 2, 1988; International Symposium on E, Kyoto, Japan, December 5–6, 1986.

14. Packer, "Protective Role of Vitamin E"; J. J. Thiele et al., "Ozone Depletes Tocopherols and Tocotrienols Topically Applied to Murine Skin," Federation of Experimental Biological Societies (letter) 401, nos. 2–3 (January 1997): 167–70.

15. P. T. Pugliese, "The Skin, Free Radicals, and Oxidative Stress," *Dermatology Nursing* 7, no. 6 (December 1995): 361–69.

16. Ibid.

17. W. Minkin, H. Cohen, and S. Frank, "Contact Dermatitis from Deodorant" (letter), *Archives of Dermatology* 107 (1973): 774–75; J. Aeling et al., "Allergic Contact Dermatitis to Vitamin E Aerosol Deodorant" (letter), *Archives of Dermatology* 108 (1973): 579–80; M. P. Goldman and M. Rapaport, "Contact Dermatitis to Vitamin E Oil," *Journal of the American Academy of Dermatology* 120 (1984): 906–8.

18. Bernard Idson, "Vitamins in Cosmetics, an Update, Part II: Vitamin E," *Drug and Cosmetic Industry,* (August 1990): 6–10.

19. F. Nachbar and H. C. Korting, "The Role of Vitamin E in Normal and Damaged Skin," *Journal of Molecular Medicine* 73, no. 1 (January 1995): 7–17.

9: VITAMIN E, SEX, AND FERTILITY

1. F. Baumbusch, G. K. Papp, and Z. S. Kopa, "Treatment for Potency Problems with Afrodor 2000," *Acta Chir Hungary* 35, nos. 1–2 (1995–96): 87–92.

2. R. K. Sharma and A. Agarwal, "Role of Reactive Oxygen Species in Male Infertility," *Urology* 48, no. 6 (December 1996): 835–50.

3. Kessopoulous et al., "A Double-Blind Randomized Placebo Crossover Controlled Trial Using the Antioxidant Vitamin E to Treat Reactive Oxygen Species Associated with Male Infertility," *Fertility and Sterility* 64, no. 4 (October 1995): 825–31.

4. D. Vezina et al., "Selenium-E Supplementation in Infertile Men. Effects on Semen Parameters and Micronutrient Levels and Dis-

tribution," *Biological Trace Elements Research* 53, nos. 1–3 (Summer 1996): 65–83.

5. R. K. Sharma and A. Agarwal, "Role of Reactive Oxygen Species."

6. Gaby et al., *Vitamin Intake and Health,* 88.

7. N. Ndiweni and J. M. Finch, "Effects of In Vitro Supplementation of Bovine Mammary Gland Macrophages and Peripheral Blood Lymphocytes with Alpha-Tocopherol and Sodium Selenite: Implications for Udder Defenses," *Veterinary Immunology and Immunopathology* 47, nos. 1–2 (July 1995): 111–21.

8. S. Renaud et al., "Influence of Vitamin E Administration on Platelet Functions in Hormonal Contraceptive Users," *Contraception* 36 (1987): 347–58.

10: VITAMIN E AGAINST AGING

1. G. T. Vatassery et al., "Changes in Vitamin E Concentrations in Human Plasma and Platelets with Age," *Journal of the American College of Nutrition* 4 (1987): 369–75.

2. D. Harman, "Aging: A Theory Based on Free Radical and Radiation Chemistry," *Journal of Geriatrics* 11 (1956): 298–300.

3. S. Kent, "Solving the Riddle of Lipofuscin's Origin May Uncover Clues to the Aging Process," *Geriatrics* 31 (1976): 128–37.

4. J. E. Poulin et al., "Vitamin E Prevents Oxidative Modification of Brain and Lymphocyte Band 3 Proteins During Aging," *Proceedings of the National Academy of Science USA* 93, no. 11 (May 28, 1996): 5600–3.

5. William Beisel, "Vitamins and the Immune System," *Annals of the New York Academy of Sciences* 587 (1990): 5–8.

6. Ibid.

7. S. N. Meydani et al., "Effect of Vitamin E Supplementation on Immune Responsiveness of Healthy Elderly Subjects," paper presented at the New York Academy of Sciences meeting: "Vitamin E: Biochemistry and Health Implications," November 1988.

8. Simin N. Meydani, "Vitamins E and B_6 and Immune Response,"

paper presented at a symposium, "Beyond Deficiency: New Views on the Function and Health Effects of Vitamins," sponsored by the New York Academy of Sciences, 1992.

9. Shantilal Shah and Ronald Johnson, "Antioxidant Vitamin A and E Status," *Nutrition Research* 9 (1989): 705–15.

10. James Anderson and Maury Breecher, *Dr. Anderson's Antioxidant, Antiaging Health Program* (New York: Carroll & Graf, 1996): 78.

11. S. A. Peters and F. J. Kelly, "Vitamin E Supplementation in Cystic Fibrosis," *Journal of Pediatric Gastroenterology and Nutrition* 22, no. 4 (May 1996): 341–45.

12. C. Jackson et al., "Vitamin E and Alzheimer's Disease in Subjects with Down's Syndrome," *Journal of Mental Deficiency Research* 32 (1988): 479–84.

13. T. Metcalfe, D. M. Bowen, and D. P. Muller, "Vitamin E Concentration in Human Brain of Patients with Alzheimer's Disease, Fetuses with Down's Syndrome, Centenarians and Controls," *Neurochemical Research* 14 (1989): 1209–12.

14. Vishwa Singh, personal communication with author, March 26, 1997.

15. Poulin et al., "Vitamin E Prevents Oxidative Modification."

16. D. B. Calne et al., "Alzheimer's Disease, Parkinson's Disease, and Motorneuron Disease: Abiotropic Interaction Between Aging and Environment?" *Lancet* 2 (1986): 1067–70.

17. J. L. Cadet et al., "Free Radicals in Tardive Dyskinesia," *Trends in Neuroscience* 9 (1986): 107–8; J. D. Grimes et al., "Antioxidant Therapy in Parkinson's Disease," *Canadian Journal of Neurology* 14 (1987): 483–87.

18. S. Fahn, "The Endogenous Toxin Hypothesis of the Etiology of Parkinson's Disease and a Pilot Trial of High-Dose Antioxidants in an Attempt to Slow the Progression of the Illness," *Annals of the New York Academy of Science* 570 (1989): 186–96.

19. J. B. Lohr et al., "Alpha Tocopherol in Tardive Dyskinesia," *Lancet* 1 (1987): 913.

20. The Parkinson Study Group, "The Effects of Tocopherol and

Deprenyl on the Progression of Disability in Early Parkinson's Disease," *New England Journal of Medicine* 328 (January 21, 1993): 176–83.

21. Ibid.

22. D. P. Muller, "Vitamin E—Its Role in Neurological Function," *Postgraduate Medicine* 62 (1986): 107–12.

23. Anthony Diplock, "The Protective Roles of Antioxidant Nutrients in Disease Prevention," *Vitamin Nutrition Information Service Backgrounder* 3, no. 1 (1992).

24. D. C. Kosegarten and J. J. Maher, "Use of Guinea Pigs as a Model to Study Galacture-Induced Cataract Formation," *Journal of Pharmacological Science* 67 (1978): 1478–79; T. M. Ferguson, R. H. Rigden, and J. R. Couch, "Cataracts in Vitamin E Deficiency, an Experimental Study in the Turkey Embryo," *Archives of Ophthalmology* 55 (1956): 346–55; P. F. Jacques et al., "Nutritional Status in Persons with and without Senile Cataract: Blood, Vitamin, and Mineral Levels," *American Journal of Clinical Nutrition* 48 (1988): 152–58.

25. J. M. Robertson, A. P. Donner, and J. R. Trevithick, "Vitamin E Intake and Risk of Cataract in Humans," *Annals of the New York Academy of Sciences* 570 (1989): 372–82.

26. P. Knekt et al., "Serum Antioxidant Vitamins and Risk of Cataract," *British Medical Journal* 305 (1992): 1392–94.

27. Johanna M. Seddon et al., "The Use of Vitamin Supplements and the Risk of Cataract Among U.S. Male Physicians," *American Journal of Public Health* 84, no. 5 (May 1994): 788–92.

28. P. F. Jacques, R. B. McGandy, and S. C. Hartz, "Antioxidant Status in Persons with and without Senile Cataract," *Archives of Ophthalmology* 106 (1988): 337–40; Robertson, Donner, and Trevithick, "Vitamin E Intake and Risk of Cataracts."

29. Julie Mares-Perlman et al., "Diet and Nuclear Lens Opacities," *American Journal of Epidemiology,* February 1995.

30. Jacques, McGandy, and Hartz, "Antioxidant Status in Persons."

31. A. Taylor, "Association Between Nutrition and Cataract," *Nutrition Review* 47 (1989): 225–34.

32. National Advisory Eye Council, *Report of the Retinal and Choroidal Diseases Panel: Vision Research: A National Plan: 1983–87,* NIH Publication 83-2471 (Washington, D.C.: U.S. Department of Health and Human Services, 1984).

33. R. Klein, B. Klein, and K. L. P. Linton, "Prevalence of Age-Related Maculopathy: The Beaver Dam Study," *Ophthalmology* 99 (1992): 933–43.

34. J. Seddon and C. Hennekens, "Vitamins, Minerals, and Macular Degeneration: Promising but Unproven Hypotheses," *Archives of Ophthalmology* 112 (February 1994): 176–77.

35. Sheila West et al., "Are Antioxidants or Supplements Protective for Age-Related Macular Degeneration?" *Archives of Ophthalmology* 112 (1994): 222–27.

36. Eye Disease Case-Control Study Group, "Antioxidant Status and Neovascular Age-Related Macular Degeneration," *Archives of Ophthalmology* 111 (January 1993): 104.

37. T. Yoskhikawa, H. Tanaka, and M. Kondo, "Effect of Vitamin E on Adjuvant Arthritis in Rats," *Biochemical Medicine* 29 (1983): 227–34.

38. G. Blankenhorn, "Clinical Efficacy of Spondyvit (Vitamin E) in Activated Arthroses. A Multicenter, Placebo-Controlled, Double-Blind Study," *Orthopedics* 124 (1986): 340–43.

39. K. H. Schmidt and W. Bayer, "Efficacy of Vitamin E as a Drug in Inflammatory Joint Disease," *Antioxidants in Therapy and Preventative Medicine,* ed. I. Emerit et al. (New York: Plenum, 1990): 147–50.

40. Singh, personal communication.

41. B. A. Watkins, H. Xu, and J. J. Turek, "Lineolate Impairs Collagen Synthesis in Primary Cultures of Avian Chondrocytes," *Proceedings of the Society for Experimental Biology in Medicine* 212, no. 2 (June 1996): 153–59; H. Xu, B. A. Watkins, and M. F. Seifert, "Vitamin E Stimulates Trabecular Bone Formation and Alters Epiphyseal Cartilage Morphometry," *Calcified Tissue International* 57, no. 4 (October 1995): 293–300.

42. Ruth Winter, *Vitamin E* (New York: Arco Publishing, 1972): 62.

43. R. Kakkar, J. S. Bains, and S. P. Sharma, "Effect of Vitamin E on Life Span, Malondialdehyde Content and Antioxidant Enzymes in Aging *Zaprionus paravittiger*," *Gerontology* 42, no. 6 (1996): 312–21.

44. K. G. Losonczy, T. B. Harris, and R. J. Havlik, "Vitamin E and Vitamin C Supplement Use and Risk of All-Cause and Coronary Heart Disease Mortality in Older Persons: The Established Populations for Epidemiologic Studies of the Elderly," *American Journal of Clinical Nutrition* 64, no. 2 (August 1996): 190–96.

45. M. F. Muldoon et al., "Serum Total Antioxidant Activity in Relative Hypo- and Hypercholesterolemia," *Free Radical Research* 25, no. 3 (September 1996): 239–45.

46. D. Harman, "Free-Radical Theory of Aging. Increasing the Functional Life Span," *Annals of the New York Academy of Science* 717 (June 30, 1994): 1–15.

11: HOW MUCH VITAMIN E DO YOU NEED?

1. M. K. Horwitt, "Interpretations of Requirements for Thiamin, Riboflavin, Niacin-Tryptophan, and Vitamin E Plus Comments on Balance Studies and Vitamin B_6," *American Journal of Clinical Nutrition* 44 (1986): 973–85.

2. *NAS-NRC Recommended Dietary Allowances,* 10th ed., (Washington, D.C.: National Academy of Sciences, 1989), 102–4.

3. Vishwa Singh, personal communcation with author, March 26, 1997.

4. Ibid.

5. Packer, "Protective Role of Vitamin E."

6. William Mergens and Hemminge Bhagavan, "Alpha Tocopherols (Vitamin E)," in *Nutrition and Cancer Prevention,* ed. Dekker, Thomas Moon, and Marc Micozzi (New York: March 1989): 331.

7. Voelker, "Recommendations for Antioxidants."

8. Paula Kurtzweil and Theresa Young, "Vitamin of the Month: Vitamin E," *FDA Consumer,* (November 1990): 31.

9. John Wallingrod, personal communication with author, March 17, 1997.

10. J. A. Lemons and M. J. Maisels, "Vitamin E—How Much Is Too Much?" *Pediatrics* 76 (1985): 625–27.

11. A. Bendich and L. J. Machlin, "Safety of Oral Intake of Vitamin E," *American Journal of Clinical Nutrition* 48 (1988): 612–19.

12. M. Briggs, "Vitamin E Supplements and Fatigue" (letter), *New England Journal of Medicine* 290 (1974): 579–80.

13. Ibid.

14. Bendich and Machlin, "Safety of Oral Intake."

15. S. Takamatsu et al., "Effects on Health of Dietary Supplementation with 100 mg d-a-Tocopheryl Acetate, Daily for Six Years," *Journal of International Medical Research* 23 (1995): 342–57.

16. M. L. Biernbaum et al., "The Effect of Supplemental Vitamin E on Serum Parameters in Diabetics, Postcoronary and Normal Subjects," *Nutrition Reports International* 31 (1985): 1171–80.

17. Bendich and Machlin, "Safety of Oral Intake"; H. Kappus and A. T. Diplock, "Tolerance and Safety of Vitamin E: A Toxicological Position Report," *Free Radical Biological Medicine* 13 (1992): 55–74.

18. Gaby et al., *Vitamin Intake and Health,* 91.

19. Bendich and Machlin, "Safety of Oral Intake."

20. M. Reilly et al., "Modulation of Oxidant Stress In Vivo in Chronic Cigarette Smokers," *Circulation* 94, no. 1 (July 1996): 19–25.

21. Ibid.

22. "American Heart Association Names Vitamin E in Year's Top 10 List," (American Heart Association news release) December 19, 1996.

23. Voelker, "Recommendations for Antioxidants."

12: VITAMIN E IN RAW, PROCESSED, AND COOKED FOOD

1. Martha Hamilton, Vitamin E Shortage Is Growing Old Fast, *Washington Post,* June 9, 1996, 1.
2. *Nutrition Business Journal* 1, no. 3 (October 1996): 16.
3. G. W. Burton and K. U. Ingold, "Vitamin E: Application of the Principles of Physical Organic Chemistry to the Exploration of Its Structure and Function," *Accounts of Chemical Research* 19 (1986): 194–201; K. U. Ingold et al., "Biokinetics of and Discrimination Between Dietary RRR and SRR-Alpha Tocopherols in the Male Rat," *Lipids* 22 (1987): 163–72.
4. *Nutrition Business Journal* 1, no. 3 (October 1996): 15–16.
5. Ibid.
6. G. W. Burton et al., "Comparison of Free Alpha-Tocopherol and Alpha-Tocopherol Acetate as Sources of Vitamin E in Rats and Humans," *Lipids* 23 (1988): 834–40. *Vitamin E Fact Book,* Veris Research and Information Service (1996): 48–50.
7. Audrey Ensminger et al., *The Concise Encyclopedia of Foods and Nutrition* (Boca Raton, Fla.: CRC Press, 1994), 1101.
8. Ibid.
9. Ibid.
10. J. B. Bauernfeind, "Tocopherols in Foods," *Vitamin E: A Comprehensive Treatise,* U.S. Dept. of Agriculture (1980): 104–17.
11. Jeffrey Blumberg, personal communication with the author, March 17, 1997.

GLOSSARY

Active immunity. Immunity produced by the body in response to stimulation by a disease-causing organism or a vaccine.

Alzheimer's disease. A deterioration of the brain with severe memory impairment.

AMD. Abbreviation for age-related macular degeneration (see MACULAR DEGENERATION).

Antioxidant. A substance that can protect another substance from oxidation. Examples are vitamins E and A.

Arteriosclerosis. Commonly known as hardening of the arteries, arteriosclerosis includes a variety of conditions that cause the artery walls to thicken and lose elasticity.

Atherosclerosis. Fatty deposits on the inner walls of the arteries.

Beta-carotene. Provitamin A. Found in all plants and in many animal tissues. It is the chief yellow-coloring matter of carrots. It is an antioxidant and is believed to play a part in immunity.

Biochemical. A substance produced by a chemical reaction in a living organism. Some can also be made in the laboratory.

Bypass surgery. A procedure to bypass the blockage or narrowing of an artery. Blockages can be bypassed using sections of normal artery or vein taken from the patient or by using synthetic tubing.

Carotenoids. Found in parsley, carrots, sweet potatoes, and most green, red, and yellow vegetables and fruits, these are vitamin A precursors that are antioxidants. There are hundreds of carotenoids in nature.

Cholesterol. Found in all body tissues, especially the brain and spinal cord, it is also present in many animal food products. It is a fatlike compound but is actually an alcohol.

Clinical trials. These are generally controlled studies involving patients. In the pharmaceutical field, companies first file an Investigational New Drug Application with the FDA to begin testing a drug's effects in people. Even if a drug is not involved, researchers are usually required to clear an experiment involving humans with an Institutional Review Board to protect the safety of participants.

Cystic fibrosis. An inherited disease of the exocrine glands, which pour secretions out of the body rather than into the blood. These include the pancreas, biliary, intestinal, and sweat glands. In this disease, thick, viscid secretions obstruct or depress the functioning of many different organs and tissues.

Cystic mastitis. The breast contains benign, usually painful, nodules and small cysts of rubbery consistency. Often frightening to women, who believe they may have a malignant lump.

Diabetes. A common disorder that occurs when the pancreas either totally stops producing insulin or does not produce enough of the hormone for the body's needs. With insulin-dependent diabetes or Type I, which occurs mainly in young people, the pancreas produces little or no insulin. Type I accounts for 5–10 percent of diabetes. In non-insulin-dependent diabetes or Type II, people over forty are usually affected. Their insulin-producing cells in the pancreas function, but the output of insulin is inadequate for the body's needs. People who have this form are usually overweight. Type II accounts for 90–95 percent of diabetes and is nearing epidemic proportions due to an increased number of older Americans, and a greater prevalence of obesity and sedentary lifestyle.

DNA. Abbreviation for deoxyribonucleic acid. A chain of molecules that contain the genetic code (blueprint) of cells.

Dopamine. 3-hydroxytyramine. An intermediate in tyrosine metabolism and the precursor of the self-produced stimulants norephinephrine and epinephrine. It is a brain chemical that initiates movement.

Double-blind clinical trial. A placebo (see) is designed to look, feel, and taste exactly like the substance being tested, so that neither the investigator nor the subjects know who is taking the active ingredient.

Enzymes. Workhorses of the cell that, without changing themselves, convert other substances such as food into products the body can use. More than a thousand different enzymes have been identified in the human body.

Epidemiological study. A study that measures the incidence of disease in large population groups and looks for associations with various genetic or environmental factors.

Epidermis. The outer portion of the skin.

Epithelium. The cellular covering of internal and external body surfaces, including the lining of vessels and small cavities. The epithelium consists of cells joined by small amounts of cementing substances and is classified according to the number of its layers and the shape of the cells.

Erythrocytes. Red blood cells, which are made in the bone marrow and transport oxygen from the lungs through the bloodstream to cells all over the body.

Esophagus. That portion of the digestive canal between the throat and stomach.

Estrogen. A hormone produced by the ovaries that is mainly responsible for female sexual characteristics. Estrogen influences bone mass by slowing or halting bone loss, improving retention of calcium by the kidneys, and improving the absorption of dietary calcium by the intestines. Estrogen is given to relieve menopausal symptoms, prevent or relieve aging changes in the vagina and urethra, and to help prevent osteoporosis—thinning of the bones.

Fatty acids. Compounds of carbon, hydrogen, and oxygen that combine with glycerol to make fats.

Fibrin. The substance that meshes blood cells in the blood-clotting mechanism. Fibrin is a body protein that hardens when blood leaves its usual channels.

Free radicals. Highly reactive molecules generated when a cell "burns" its food with oxygen to fuel life processes. Free radicals act like "loose cannons," rolling around and damaging cells. This damage is thought to be a first step in cancer development. Antioxidants such as vitamin E and a number of phytochemicals found in food can suppress free-radical cell damage.

Gene. The smallest genetic unit of a chromosome. It is a piece of DNA that contains the hereditary information for the production of a protein.

Glucose. Sugar that occurs naturally in blood, grapes, and corn. A source of energy for animals and plants.

Gram. Unit of the metric system that equals 0.035 ounce.

HDL. The abbreviation for high-density lipoprotein. HDL is believed to pick up excess cholesterol in the blood and help the body eliminate it.

Hypoglycemia. Low blood sugar—the opposite of diabetes.

Hypothalamus. Brain control area involved in emotions, movements, and eating. Less than the size of a peanut and weighing a quarter of an ounce, this small area deep within the brain also oversees appetite, blood pressure, sexual behavior, and sleep and sends orders to the pituitary gland.

Immunity. Body mechanisms create immunities to disease germs and foreign substances. These are the following basics:

- *Acquired* (*active*) results from having recovered from a disease or from being given an immunizing vaccine or serum.

- *Inherent* (*innate*) is the type with which one is born.
- *Local* involves tissues or areas or organs of the body that manifest an acquired or natural immunity against infection. Your intestinal tract, for example, is immune to infection from many of the bacteria that live and grow within it.
- *Natural* results from recovery from an illness or from innate resistance to a particular bacteria or virus.

Impotence. Inability of the male to have a penile erection and perform the sexual act. Impotence is a problem of delivery rather than of production of sperm.

Infarct. An area of dead tissue resulting from a blockage of its blood supply. This frequently occurs in coronary thrombosis, the type of heart attack in which a clot blocks the coronary artery.

Insulin. A hormone produced by the islet cells of the pancreas gland, essential for metabolism. Insulin is used in the treatment of diabetes.

Intermittent claudication. Pain in the calf muscles and limping due to inadequate blood supply.

Ischemia. Local deficiency of blood supply, due to obstruction or spasms of an artery.

IU. Abbreviation for international unit, used to express the biological activity of vitamin E. Up until 1980, the RDA for vitamin E was expressed in IUs. However, in 1980, the term *tocopherol equivalent* (TE) was used to express the RDA for vitamin E. By this system, 1 mg of d-alpha tocopherol, the most active of the naturally occurring forms of the vitamin, is equivalent to 1.49 IU vitamin E. Many still use IU instead of mg, as we did throughout this book.

LDL. Abbreviation for low-density lipoprotein, which is believed to collect cholesterol in the blood and deposit it in the cells.

Leukocytes. White blood cells, which fight disease.

Lipid. A fatty substance found in food and in the body. In the body, lipids are sources of stored energy, but they can also build up within the blood vessels causing blockages. Triglycerides are lipids.

Lipid peroxidation. Oxidation of fat, leading to decomposition.

Low blood sugar. See HYPOGLYCEMIA.

Lymph. A liquid found within the lymphatic vessels (see), containing white blood cells and some red blood cells. These cells, collected from tissues throughout the body, flow in the lymphatic vessels through the lymph nodes, and eventually into the blood. Lymph is an important part of the body's ability to fight infections and diseases.

Lymphatic vessels. A bodywide network of channels, similar to the blood vessels, that transport lymph to the immune organs and into the bloodstream.

Lymphocytes. Small white blood cells produced in the lymphoid organs and paramount in the immune system.

Macrophage. A large and versatile immune cell that acts as a devouring cell, antigen-presenting cell, and an important source of immune secretions.

Macular degeneration. An area of the retina near the optic nerve at the back of the eye that distinguishes fine detail at the center of the field of vision. Degeneration occurs when the small blood vessels of the eye become constricted and hardened and there is insufficient blood supply to the macula. It is strongly age-related with prevalence rising to 22 percent by age seventy-five.

Mastitis. Inflammation of the breasts, from bacterial infection or other causes.

Metabolism. The chemical processes in living organisms that allow growth, production of energy, and the maintenance of vital functions of living. Carbohydrates are the most important nutrients for metabolism with fats second and proteins third.

Mg. Abbreviation for milligram, which is a thousandth of a gram (see).

Molecule. The smallest amount of a specific chemical substance that can exist alone.

Mutation. A permanent change in the genetic material that will be passed on to a new generation of cells.

Myelin. White fatty material that covers most nerves, similar to insulation covering wires.

Nitrosamines. Cancer-causing agents formed in the gastrointestinal tract from reactions in which nitrites and nitrates combine with amines, organic compounds present in the body.

Oxidation. The process of combining with oxygen. When combined with fat, oxygen makes the fat rancid. Oxidation provides needed energy for life, but also produces free radicals (see).

Oxygen. An odorless gas necessary for life. The air we breathe is 20 percent oxygen. The oxygen we breathe is carried to all tissues by the red blood cells.

Parkinson's disease. Chronic neurologic disease characterized by tremors, rigidity, and an abnormal gait.

Placebo. An inert or innocuous substance given in place of medication.

Plasma. The fluid portion of the blood or lymph, which carries in solution a wide range of ions, minerals, vitamins, antibodies, proteins, enzymes, and/or other essential substances.

Platelet. A component of blood that plays an important role in blood coagulation.

Platelet aggregation. A clumping together of platelets that may lead to a blood clot or plaques that block arteries.

Polyunsaturated. Plant fats that are liquid at room temperature. They have more bonds between carbon atoms than do saturated (see) fats and can take on additional hydrogen atoms; thus they are more chemically active and it is believed they can cause a depletion of vitamin E.

Precursor. A substance turned into another active, or more mature, substance by a biologic process. Beta-carotene is a precursor of vitamin A because the body can use it to make vitamin A.

Prostacyclin. A derivative of prostaglandins (see) that is a natural inhibitor of platelet aggregation and is a blood vessel dilator.

Prostaglandins. PGA. PGB. PGC. PGD. A group of extremely potent hormonelike substances present in many tissues. More than sixteen are known, with effects such as dilating or constricting blood vessels, stimulating intestinal or bronchial smooth muscle, uterine stimulation, antagonism to hormones, and influencing metabolism of fat. Various prostaglandins in the body can cause fever, inflammation, and headache. Prostaglandins or drugs that affect prostaglandins are used medically to induce labor, prevent and treat peptic ulcers, control high blood pressure, treat bronchial asthma, and induce delayed menstruation. Aspirin and other NSAIDs tend to inhibit prostaglandin production.

Randomized. Drugs are assigned to patients in no particular order during testing of the effects of a pharmaceutical.

Red blood cells. See ERYTHROCYTES.

Restless leg syndrome (RLS). Occurs at bedtime and is described as "running in bed." Symptoms are vague, with twitching and muscular discomfort.

Retina. The light-receiving cells at the back of the eye. Hundreds of thousands of nerve endings in the retina merge into the optic nerve, which conveys impulses to the "seeing" part of the brain at the back of your head.

RNA. Ribonucleic acid, which is found in the cytoplasm and also in the nucleus of some cells. One function of RNA is to direct the manufacture of proteins.

Saturated fats. Animal fats, solid at room temperature. Saturation refers to the ratio of hydrogen atoms to carbon atoms. Saturated fats have been accused of contributing to atherosclerosis (see). Also see POLYUNSATURATED.

Sedentary. Sitting still much of the time.

Thrombus. A blood clot that forms within the heart or a blood vessel and remains attached to its point of origin.

Triglycerides. Sweet fatty substances, the result of digestion. They contain three fatty acids combined with one molecule of glycerol.

Ultraviolet. Radiation from sunlight that reaches the earth's surface. Ultraviolet A rays have longer wavelengths than ultraviolet B and are of lower energy. Approximately a thousand times more ultraviolet A energy than ultraviolet B energy is needed to produce skin redness or sunburn. However, because the solar energy reaching the earth's surface contains ten to one hundred times more ultraviolet A than ultraviolet B, ultraviolet A can have significant effects on the body.

Vitamin A. Exists in two main forms in nature: as retinol, found only in animal sources, and as certain carotenoids, found mainly in yellow fruits and vegetables. Carotenoids are only one-third as potent as retinol. High levels of vitamin E can block the conversion of beta-carotene into vitamin A. It is an antioxidant (see).

Vitamin C. Helps to form the connective tissue collagen; promotes wound healing; keeps blood vessels strong; enhances iron absorption. It is an antioxidant (see).

Vitamins. Chemical compounds that are vital for growth, health, metabolism, and physical and mental well-being. Some vitamins aid enzymes, the workhorses of the body that perform chemical reactions. Other vitamins form parts of hormones—the directors sent out from glands to turn on or off other organs. There are two basic types of vitamins—fat soluble and water soluble. The fat soluble, such as vitamin A, can accumulate in the body and cause problems if taken in excessive amounts. The water-soluble vitamins, such as vitamin C, cannot be stored to any great degree and must be obtained through foods.

Wheat germ. The golden germ of the wheat, about 2.5 percent of the whole wheat kernel, is high in vitamin E. The germ contains thiamin, riboflavin, and pyridoxine.

White blood cells. See LEUKOCYTES.

INDEX

Conversion Chart

EQUIVALENT IMPERIAL AND METRIC MEASUREMENT

Americans use standard containers, the 8-ounce cup and a tablespoon that takes exactly 16 level fillings to fill that cup level. Measuring by cup makes it very difficult to give weight equivalents, as a cup of densely packed butter will weigh considerably more than a cup of flour. The easiest way therefore to deal with cup measurements is to take the amount by volume rather than by weight. Thus the equation reads: *1 cup = 240 ml = 8 fl. oz.   1/2 cup = 120 ml = 4 fl. oz.*

SOLID MEASURES

U.S. and Imperial Measures		*Metric Measures*	
ounces	pounds	grams	kilos
1		28	
2		56	
3½		100	
4	¼	112	
5		140	
6		168	
8	½	225	
9		250	¼
12	¾	340	
16	1	450	
18		500	½
20	1¼	560	
24	1½	675	
27		750	¾
28	1¾	780	
32	2	900	
36	2¼	1000	1
40	2½	1100	
48	3	1350	
54		1500	1½
64	4	1800	

U.S. and Imperial Measures		Metric Measures	
ounces	pounds	grams	kilos
72	4½	2000	2
80	5	2250	2¼
90		2500	2½
100	6	2800	2¾

LIQUID MEASURES

Fluid ounces	U.S.	Imperial	Milliliters
	1 teaspoon	1 teaspoon	5
¼	2 teaspoons	1 dessertspoon	10
½	1 tablespoon	1 tablespoon	14
1	2 tablespoons	2 tablespoons	28
2	¼ cup	4 tablespoons	56
4	½ cup		110
5		¼ pint or 1 gill	140
6	¾ cup		170
8	1 cup		225
9			250
10	1¼ cups	½ pint	280
12	1½ cups		340
15		3/4 pint	420
16	2 cups		450
18	2¼ cups		500
20	2½ cups	1 pint	560
24	3 cups		675
25		1¼ pints	700
27	3½ cups		750
30	3¾ cups	1½ pints	840
32	4 cups or 1 quart		900
35		1¾ pints	980
36	4½ cups		1000
40	5 cups	2 pints or 1 quart	1120
48	6 cups		1350
50		2½ pints	1400
60	7½ cups	3 pints	1680
64	8 cups or 2 quarts		1800
72	9 cups		2000